T0292400

Veterinary Business and Enterprise: Theoretical Foundations and Practical Cases

Content Strategist: Robert Edwards
Content Development Specialist: Veronika Watkins/Carole McMurray
Project Manager: Kiruthiga Kasthuriswamy/Beula Christopher
Designer/Design Direction: Christian Bilbow
Illustration Manager: Jennifer Rose
Illustrator: Richard Tibbitts

Veterinary Business and Enterprise: Theoretical Foundations and Practical Cases

Edited by

Colette Henry

Foreword by

The Right Honourable The Lord Ballyedmond OBE

Chairman, Norbrook Laboratories Ltd

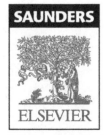

SAUNDERS

ELSEVIER

Edinburgh London New York Oxford Philadelphia St Louis Sydney Toronto 2014

SAUNDERS
ELSEVIER

© 2014, Elsevier Ltd. All rights reserved.

No part of this publication may be reproduced or transmitted in any form or by any means, electronic or mechanical, including photocopying, recording, or any information storage and retrieval system, without permission in writing from the publisher. Details on how to seek permission, further information about the Publisher's permissions policies and our arrangements with organizations such as the Copyright Clearance Center and the Copyright Licensing Agency, can be found at our website: www.elsevier.com/permissions.

This book and the individual contributions contained in it are protected under copyright by the Publisher (other than as may be noted herein).

ISBN 978-0-7020-5012-1

British Library Cataloguing in Publication Data
A catalogue record for this book is available from the British Library

Library of Congress Cataloging in Publication Data
A catalog record for this book is available from the Library of Congress

---

Notices

Knowledge and best practice in this field are constantly changing. As new research and experience broaden our understanding, changes in research methods, professional practices, or medical treatment may become necessary.

Practitioners and researchers must always rely on their own experience and knowledge in evaluating and using any information, methods, compounds, or experiments described herein. In using such information or methods they should be mindful of their own safety and the safety of others, including parties for whom they have a professional responsibility.

With respect to any drug or pharmaceutical products identified, readers are advised to check the most current information provided (i) on procedures featured or (ii) by the manufacturer of each product to be administered, to verify the recommended dose or formula, the method and duration of administration, and contraindications. It is the responsibility of practitioners, relying on their own experience and knowledge of their patients, to make diagnoses, to determine dosages and the best treatment for each individual patient, and to take all appropriate safety precautions.

To the fullest extent of the law, neither the Publisher nor the authors, contributors, or editors, assume any liability for any injury and/or damage to persons or property as a matter of products liability, negligence or otherwise, or from any use or operation of any methods, products, instructions, or ideas contained in the material herein.

---

your source for books, journals and multimedia in the health sciences

www.elsevierhealth.com

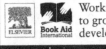
Working together to grow libraries in developing countries

www.elsevier.com • www.bookaid.org

The Publisher's policy is to use paper manufactured from sustainable forests

Printed in China

Contents

PART 1 Theoretical foundations

PART 2 Practical cases

Website

The additional online resources can be found on **www.enterprisingvet.com**

The website includes:

- Video introduction from, and interview with, the author
- Key learning objectives
- Case study questions and assignments

Sarah Baillie BVSc, MSc(IT), PhD, MRCVS is Professor of Veterinary Education at the School of Veterinary Sciences, University of Bristol, UK. She was a veterinarian in private practice for 20 years, where her interests included cattle health and production, small-animal surgery and business development. She is currently responsible for curriculum development at Bristol, and her research interests include informal lifelong learning, business skills, transition into practice and mental health. She is involved in designing and evaluating haptic (virtual, yet touchable) simulators.

Christopher J. Brown PhD is the University of Hertfordshire's Business School Knowledge Transfer Leader, as a consequence of which he is actively involved in business and community engagement. His thirty years of experience in manufacturing, transport and defence have proved valuable in developing relationships between business and the university. His research interests in sustainability, innovation and business models help in his understanding and interpretation of business challenges and issues. Parasol Kennels is just one example of the type of collaboration and mentoring project with which the university engages.

Martin A. Cake BSc, BVMS, PhD is Associate Professor and Associate Dean of Teaching and Learning within the School of Veterinary and Biomedical Sciences, Murdoch University, Western Australia, where he teaches veterinary anatomy and professional life skills to veterinary undergraduates. His research lies mostly in osteoarthritis and connective tissue biology, but he also has a keen interest in education and curriculum development. He recently initiated a systematic review of evidence for the importance of non-technical veterinary graduate attributes.

Catherine Coates MA(Ed), PGCert BusAdmin, PGCE, BA(Hons), DipIT (Open), CVPM is a Teaching Fellow at the University of Bristol, School of Veterinary Science. Catherine started her career at the university as an administrator within the Division of Companion Animal Studies, managing the finances of the division's small-animal veterinary referral hospital and two first-opinion practices. She was appointed Lecturer in Veterinary Practice Management at the university in 2003 and was promoted to Teaching Fellow in 2008. Catherine lectures on a variety of management topics, and is a Unit and Element Organiser responsible for designing programme content, delivery and assessment both on the veterinary and veterinary nursing undergraduate programmes at Bristol.

Claire Denny BVetMed, MRCVS graduated from the Royal Veterinary College in 2010 with Honours. During her final year she was involved in research exploring the use of case studies as an educational tool to teach Day One business skills to undergraduate veterinary students. For this work she was awarded the London BioScience Innovation Centre Prize. After graduating she spent a year working as a houseman in a busy practice in the Midlands. She now works in a small-animal practice in Kent.

Andrew Donaldson BSc, MSc, PhD is a Senior Lecturer in the School of Architecture, Planning and Landscape, Newcastle University. He has a background in natural and social sciences. His research focuses on the framing and management of biological and natural risks. He has been a leading figure in the development of social scientific studies of animal health issues and agricultural biosecurity since 2001, and has acted as an expert advisor to the National Audit Office on animal health policy.

Brian Faulkner BSc(Hons), BVM&S, MBA, MSc (Psych), GPcert(SAM), GPcert(B&PS), MRCVS is an experienced veterinary clinician and practice management consultant, having worked in over 100 veterinary practices over the past 18 years. He set up, developed and sold a cluster of veterinary practices in the UK between 2002 and 2009. He was voted the Petplan UK Vet of the Year in 2008. He is Honorary Lecturer in Veterinary Entrepreneurship at Nottingham University and the Vice Chair of the European School of Veterinary Post Graduate Studies in Business and Professional Studies. He is particularly interested in the mindsets which foster the confidence to excel within veterinary practice and is a regular speaker at various UK veterinary conferences on these subjects. He is also an Officer at the Society of Practising Veterinary Surgeons.

Adele Feakes BVSc Hons (Melb 1983), GCertHEd is Lecturer Veterinary (Practice) Management in the School of Animal and Veterinary Sciences at the University of Adelaide, South Australia. Her experience as a veterinarian includes working in animal emergency practice, in small-animal practice, as a production animal and equine veterinarian while a principal (for 24 years) of a successful rural veterinary practice in South Australia, as an On Plant Veterinary Officer with AQIS (Australian Quarantine Inspection Service) and as a member of the Board of Directors of the Australian Veterinary Association. Adele's research and teaching interests are in pedagogy for development of an enterprising mind-set for veterinary students and also in the development of entrepreneurial psychometric instruments for veterinary and students of other health sciences. Her research question is "What factors contribute to the development of career and entrepreneurial intent and capability in veterinary students?".

James Gazzard BSc(Hons), PhD, MBA, PgCert(Vet Ed) is Professor of Workforce Futures in the Faculty of Medicine and Health Sciences, University of East Anglia. He previously led the enterprise education portfolio in Bio-Veterinary Science at the Royal Veterinary College. He coordinated the veterinary business elective modules, the Innovets extramural study programme and the business curriculum for veterinary scientists. James has also held various roles focused on enterprise, innovation and training at GlaxoSmithKline, Cranfield School of Management and the Medical Research Council.

Colette Henry BA(Hons), MBA, PhD, FHEA, FRSA, FISBE is an Adjunct Professor at Tromsø University Business School, Norway. She held the Norbrook Chair in Business and Enterprise at the Royal Veterinary College (RVC), University of London, where she led the BVetMed veterinary undergraduate business curriculum and designed the business research agenda. Colette was previously Head of Department of Business Studies at Dundalk Institute of Technology, and Commercial Trader at Commercial Metals Belgium. She has published widely on entrepreneurship education and training, programme evaluation, women's entrepreneurship and the creative industries, and more recently on veterinary entrepreneurship education and gender. Colette is the founding editor of the *International Journal of Gender and Entrepreneurship* (IJGE), and co-series editor of Routledge's Masters Series in Entrepreneurship.

Lynne V. Hill MVB, MBA, MRCVS is Chief Executive Officer of Langford Veterinary Services Ltd at the University of Bristol. A Veterinary Science graduate of Trinity College Dublin, she worked in mixed animal practice for 12 years in both Lancashire and Northern Ireland before primarily working with small animals. She then worked for an international pet food company as European Marketing Manager, and subsequently moved to the Royal Veterinary College to become Director of the Queen Mother Hospital. Lynne became Head of the Department of Clinical Services, running their equine and small-animal clinics as well as their diagnostic labs. Lynne is a former President of the Royal College of Veterinary Surgeons and the first woman President of the British Small Animal Veterinary Association.

Fionn Latooij BSc(Hons) VetPath is a final year Veterinary Medicine student at the Royal Veterinary College (RVC). He has led the RVC chapter of the Veterinary Business Management Association (VBMA) for two consecutive years and has been closely involved with the development of the business, enterprise and management curriculum. He has also helped stimulate further student interest and visiting lecturer contacts for the RVC in that time.

Philip Lowe MA, MSc, MPhil, OBE, AcSS is the Duke of Northumberland Professor of Rural Economy at the Centre for Rural Economy, School of Agriculture, Food and Rural Development, University of Newcastle. He is also Director of the Rural Economy and Land Use (RELU) Programme of the UK Research Councils. He has been a leading figure in the development of interdisciplinary rural studies in the UK. He has played an active role in rural policy development at the national and European levels and in the north of England. For his contribution to the rural economy he was awarded an OBE in 2003. He was Chairman of the Vets and Veterinary Services Working Group (2007–9) and produced the influential report to the government's 'Unlocking Potential: A Report on veterinary expertise in food animal production' in 2009.

Andrew Morton BA(Hons), DipN is a Fellow of the Chartered Institute of Marketing and Chartered Marketer. He is a highly experienced and skilled marketer. His career includes senior agency posts and senior management client-side experience working with major international brands. He is currently working as an Associate Lecturer in Digital Marketing, Marketing Management, New Product Development and Business Leadership at Plymouth University Business School and Exeter University.

Liz Mossop BVM&S, MMed Sci (Clin Ed), PhD, MAcadMEd, MRCVS is Associate Professor of Veterinary Education and Sub-Dean for Teaching, Learning and Assessment at School of Veterinary Medicine and Science, University of Nottingham. Liz worked in mixed/equine practice for several years before becoming interested in education. She is a foundation member of staff at Nottingham Veterinary School and holds a PhD in Veterinary Education. Her thesis focuses on veterinary professionalism. She has a Lord Dearing award for outstanding teaching and delivers across a range of subjects, with a focus on professional skills.

Jeremy Phillipson BSc, MPhil is based at the School of Agriculture, Food and Rural Development, Centre for Rural Economy, Newcastle University. He is Assistant Director of the UK Research Councils' Rural Economy and Land Use Programme (Relu), an interdisciplinary research programme spanning the social and natural sciences (funded by ESRC, BBSRC, NERC, DEFRA and the Scottish Government). He has expertise on knowledge transfer processes, interdisciplinary research policies and practices, and participatory methods of knowledge exchange with non-scientific stakeholders. Jeremy is coordinator of Landbridge, a knowledge exchange network for rural professionals and was Principal Investigator of the ESRC 'Science in the Field' project discussed in Chapter 9. Jeremy is a member of the DECC/DEFRA Social Science Expert Panel, Land Use Fellow of the Living With Environmental Change Partnership, and a Board member of the Scottish Government RESAS Strategic Research Board.

Amy Proctor PhD is a Research Associate at the School of Agriculture, Food and Rural Development, Centre for Rural Economy, Newcastle University. She is an experienced social scientist with expertise in the fields of knowledge and expertise, and processes of knowledge exchange. As the principal researcher for 'Science in the Field', an ESRC-funded project investigating the field expertise of specialist advisors, her work has explored the role of field advisors, including vets, as knowledge brokers between institutional science, rural policy and land management practitioners. She has developed a research portfolio on veterinary expertise including contributing to a landmark series in the *Philosophical Transactions of the Royal Society* and the *Veterinary Record*, and is contributing to the RVC-led 'Advanced Training Partnership in Intensive Livestock Health and Production' programme.

Susan M. Rhind BVMS, PhD, FRCPath, FHEA, MRCVS is Chair of Veterinary Medical Education, Director of Veterinary Teaching and Head of the Veterinary Medical Education Research Division at the Royal (Dick) School of Veterinary Studies, University of Edinburgh. Her main teaching areas are in general and systems pathology. Her current research is focused on veterinary medical education, where her interests include assessment, feedback, e-learning and factors affecting transition into practice.

Robert Smith MA, PhD is a Reader in Entrepreneurship and Leadership, and the SIPR Lecturer in Leadership and Management at the Aberdeen Business School, Robert Gordon University, Aberdeen, Scotland. His primary research focus is on study of entrepreneurship in different settings and applications including the socially constructed nature of entrepreneurship, entrepreneurial identity, semiotics, narrative and storytelling in organizations, including small and family business. He has published over 70 journal articles and book chapters to date, many of which have narrative themes. His policing research interests include criminal entrepreneurship, the links between organized crime groups and business, entrepreneurial policing, community policing, police intelligence and rural policing. Robert is an ex-police officer who retired with 25 years' service to concentrate on his academic career.

Jane Taylor BA(Hons) has over 17 years of multi-sector, multi-discipline marketing experience. During her career she has worked for both international and national advertising and marketing agencies, and as European Advertising Manager for global retailers

TK Maxx, and in charge of new business and marketing for Stanton Williams Architects. Jane ran Flint Creative Solutions – part of BLM Media – for two years, and was responsible for a host of award-winning creative campaigns including *Maxim Magazine*'s 'Little Black Book' and twice IPA winner for 'Monsanto RoundUp'. Jane ran her own consultancy 'marketing Jem' between 2006 and 2009 before starting a family. Jane is now a sole trader working as Marketing Director for the Parasol Group; as copywriter for Foresite SPA; and as marketing consultant and copywriter for Finkernagel Ross Architects.

Lorna Treanor BSc(Hons), BLegSc, PgDip, FRSA, is a Lecturer in Management at the Ulster Business School, University of Ulster. Lorna is completing her doctoral research exploring gender-related barriers to women's business ownership and leadership within the veterinary profession. Lorna is Chair and co-founder of the Gender and Enterprise Network, a special-interest group of the Institute of Small Business and Entrepreneurship (ISBE), of which Lorna is also a Board member.

Martin Whiting BSc, BVetMed, MA, MRCVS, FRSA is a postgraduate researcher in the Department of Production and Population Health at the Royal Veterinary College (RVC), University of London. He graduated from RVC in 2006; he also holds a degree in philosophy and a Masters in medical ethics and law, both awarded from King's College London. After a short time in general veterinary practice, followed by an internship at a specialist small-animal hospital, Martin returned to the Royal Veterinary College to undertake a PhD in veterinary ethics and law. Martin teaches veterinary ethics and law to RVC's BVetMed students, and also teaches on the graduate diploma in nursing courses. His main interests are in veterinary ethics and law and the regulation of the veterinary profession.

Izzy Warren Smith OBE, PhD, FRSA is Principal Lecturer in Rural Economics and Entrepreneurship at Harper Adams University College, Shropshire. She is also Visiting Research Fellow at Manchester Metropolitan University Business School. Her expertise lies in assessment of the practical outworking of entrepreneurship in rural businesses. In response to her research into rural female entrepreneurship she founded WiRE (women in Rural Enterprise), a successful networking organization for female entrepreneurs with a database of over 10 000 members. For this work she received the Prowess award for 'Outstanding Contribution to Female Entrepreneurship' and 'Midlander of the Year'. Harper Adams was also given the Queens Award for its work with rural businesses.

Diane Whatling DipVN, DipHR is a Diploma Veterinary Nurse and is Practice Manager for the University of Adelaide's Companion Animal Health Centre in South Australia. She also has a Diploma in Human Resources, Business Management and Workplace training and Assessment. Diane has over thirty years' experience in small-animal practice, providing her with opportunities to own and develop an innovative small-animal practice. She was also the first recipient of a Diploma in Veterinary Nursing in South Australia, and has achieved several industry awards in business and practice management, including Veterinary Nurse of the Year in 1981. Diane spent five years as a Territory Manager for Royal Canin, and has also worked with the Australian Veterinary Association. She is currently involved in lecturing to students in marketing, human resources and daily operations of veterinary practice.

Acknowledgements

The editor is grateful to students of the Royal Veterinary College (RVC) – particularly the BVetMed years 3, 4 and 5 classes of 2011/12 – and to RVC staff and external colleagues who kindly helped with the extensive reviewing process for this book. Sincere thanks are also due to the chapter authors and their various interviewees and case subjects, without whose cooperation the production of this text would not have been possible. A special thank you to Fionn Latooij – BVetMed final year student at RVC – for compiling and leading the web-based interviews with the editor. The editor also wishes to thank the Elsevier team for their invaluable technical and professional support during the course of developing this book. Finally, the editor gratefully acknowledges the support of Norbrook Laboratories Ltd for their generous sponsorship of the project through the Norbrook Chair in Business and Enterprise at the Royal Veterinary College.

The veterinary business landscape has changed significantly in recent years. At the global level, there has been a decrease in the number of livestock and farm holdings, prompting a reduction in the demand for large-animal veterinary work. In parallel, there has been considerable growth in small-animal veterinary practice, which, not surprisingly, has created increased competition amongst veterinary practices. In some areas, small independent practices have been replaced by branded veterinary groups or joint venture partnerships, signalling a radical change to the traditional veterinary business model. In addition, corporate practices are growing in number, taking an increasing share of the companion animal market, and introducing sophisticated marketing and promotion strategies. Collectively, such changes have prompted veterinary surgeons to realize that a veterinary practice is, essentially, a small business enterprise and, as such, needs to engage in effective business strategies if it is to survive in the long term.

The dynamic and highly competitive veterinary business landscape that we are currently witnessing has also led veterinary educators to recognize that there is a significant skills gap in business and management competencies amongst their students. Indeed, this skills gap is acknowledged beyond the role of the practice manager, with recognition that professionals working within the wider veterinary sector – including those operating in the bioscience, pharmaceuticals and pet food industries, as well as veterinary advisors working in government departments – also need to acquire business and enterprise skills.

This textbook is unique in that it combines both the theory and practice of veterinary enterprise to help enhance students' understanding of veterinary business management. While the theory chapters provide students with critical underpinning business knowledge, the case study chapters offer valuable practical insights into the challenges faced by veterinary business managers. There is also a considerable variety of perspective in this book, with contributions from across a number of UK and international veterinary schools, including the Royal Veterinary College at the University of London, the University of Nottingham, University of Bristol and University of Edinburgh, as well as Murdoch and Adelaide veterinary schools in Australia. The theory chapters explore important topics of contemporary relevance to veterinary scholars, and the case studies highlight specific business challenges across a range of veterinary practice types for students to address as part of their veterinary business learning. Finally, the online component of the book, which facilitates veterinary students' increasingly heavy workload by delivering supporting materials, encourages learners to delve into their creative problem-solving abilities to find innovative solutions to real veterinary business problems.

It is incumbent on 21st-century veterinary educators to ensure that future graduates are equipped with the relevant skills and abilities not only to enhance their own employability, but also to make a real and meaningful contribution to the veterinary sector – one that goes beyond the clinical dimensions of the profession. Teaching business and enterprise at the undergraduate level has never been more important. Veterinary students need to have a more holistic understanding of the wider veterinary sector, be aware of the many changes taking place therein, and appreciate exactly how such changes will impact on the particular veterinary enterprise in which they will work in the future. This book is a step toward achieving this goal.

The Right Honourable The Lord Ballyedmond OBE
Chairman, Norbrook Laboratories Ltd

The Editor was deeply saddened to learn of the death of Lord Ballyedmond on 13th March 2014. As founder and Chairman of Norbrook Laboratories, Lord Ballyedmond was passionate about embedding entrepreneurship in veterinary curricula, and encouraging veterinary students to be entrepreneurial. With his passing, the veterinary business community has lost a true innovator and entrepreneur, someone who, in his own words, was 'elated by success and educated by failure.'

Introduction

Colette Henry

Business and enterprise, although now well established as taught disciplines in their own right, are still relatively new phenomena within veterinary scholarship. Current veterinary education curricula, as expected, are dominated by clinical content and balanced with ethical and legal teaching input relevant to the profession. Despite recognition that veterinary graduates need to have both an awareness and an understanding of the wider business dimensions of veterinary practice, as articulated, for example, by Lowe (2009), and highlighted as a professional competence requirement by the Royal College of Veterinary Surgeons (RCVS, 2006), research shows that not all veterinary schools provide business training in their undergraduate programmes (Henry, 2011). At a broader level, there is consensus that business and enterprise skills make a significant contribution to graduate employability across discipline areas (HEA, 2005) and, in this regard, veterinary graduates are no exception (Henry and Treanor, 2010, 2012).

This textbook was designed as a learning tool to support veterinary business educators in their efforts to embed business and enterprise into veterinary undergraduate curricula. Its aim is to provide students with a valuable learning platform that comprises both underpinning theory and related practical scenarios contextualized within the 'real' veterinary business world. Drawing on the expertise of both national and international veterinary educators and researchers, the text also helps address the current dearth of veterinary business educational materials, while at the same time building on and, indeed, complementing some of the contemporary veterinary practice management texts currently available (see, for example, Jerving-Back and Back,

2007; Shilcock and Stutchfield, 2008). The review questions provided at the end of each of the theory chapters, along with the case questions and team assignments accessible through the companion website, should also complement veterinary educators' own business and enterprise lecture material, thus enhancing the collective student learning experience.

The textbook is strategically divided into two parts. Following this introductory chapter, and by way of laying the foundation for the rest of the book, Part I introduces veterinary students to a range of theories and concepts relevant to veterinary business and enterprise. In chapter 2, Martin Cake, Susan Rhind and Sarah Baillie present a systematic and comprehensive literature review of both perceptions of and evidence for the importance of business skills to the success of veterinary graduates. Their review reveals that 'business skills' are included as a core domain in all published competence frameworks, although there is some ambiguity about the use of business skills terminology. In studies focusing on stakeholder perceptions of importance, business skills were consistently rated of relatively low importance when Likert-scale rating surveys were used, although they rated higher when free text data were analysed. In contrast, however, surveys of perceived competence suggested business skills were one of the weakest competences in new graduates, with this being acutely perceived as a deficiency by both graduates and employers. As a result of their review, the authors offer a number of recommendations to help veterinary schools and educators deal with this issue.

Chapter 3, by Liz Mossop, explores the concept of clinical leadership, and discusses the various skills

© 2014, Elsevier Ltd.

and behaviours necessary to become an effective leader within the veterinary profession. The rationale for the chapter is based on the fact that veterinary surgeons need to consider the development of professional skills with a particular focus on leadership. Veterinary practice teams can be complex, and require strong leadership skills in order to deliver effective clinical care. Management may differ from leadership, in that management can be more authoritarian. However, in veterinary practice there is often overlap between managers and leaders, and these differences may not be overt. Clinical leadership is therefore an important concept to consider, especially when implementing the requirements of the RCVS regarding clinical governance. Most importantly, leadership training needs to begin at undergraduate level but continue throughout a veterinary professional's career.

The leadership theme is continued by Brian Faulkner in chapter 4, which highlights the importance of both leadership and management as valuable commodities in veterinary businesses. The chapter aims to provide students with valuable insights into the variety of models that have been used to capture leadership and management concepts within other business and political arenas. The differences between management and leadership are highlighted, with 'leaders' and 'managers' presented as two distinct modes of operating, and with entirely different levels of focus and scope, ranging from the more externally observable or 'tangible' dimensions of leadership, as described in the traits, skills and styles approaches, to the more intangible or psychological level, as articulated in the transformational and cultural models. The chapter concludes that veterinary leadership is important, and that some forms of leadership can indeed be learnt.

Chapter 5, by Lorna Treanor and Martin Whiting, introduces veterinary students to the ethical management of people and practices, highlighting the knowledge and skills that employers and RCVS expect from new graduates, while also providing an insight into what they might expect as employees. Human resource management (HRM) practice within veterinary businesses is discussed, with special consideration given to the motivation, training and development of all practice staff including veterinary nurses. Key theories and concepts of ethics, professionalism and management are introduced to students, with both good and poor practice examples used to illustrate possible practical issues that may arise in the workplace.

In chapter 6, Robert Smith and Martin Whiting explore the highly controversial yet important issue of criminal enterprise within the veterinary sector. The chapter draws on case evidence to focus on the illegal trade in veterinary medicines, presenting this as a contemporary example of criminal entrepreneurship. The authors highlight the hidden and often denied nature of this illegal trade, alongside its huge negative impact on the veterinary sector in terms of both ethics and revenues. Interestingly, the chapter draws parallels between the stereotypical images of veterinarians and entrepreneurs, both of which are socially constructed as 'heroes'. The authors conclude that there is a need for veterinarians, both individually and collectively, to be vigilant so as to prevent industry outsiders or organized criminals from taking over black market opportunities. There is also value in educating and training veterinarians in how to spot and deal with examples of criminal entrepreneurship.

Chapter 7 by Andrew Morton introduces veterinary students to the concept of marketing. Effective marketing has increasingly been seen as one of the main drivers for long-term sustainable growth and, as such, has required greater investment in time and money. Additionally, recent changes in consumer behaviour and market conditions have resulted in far greater risks for veterinary practice owners and managers. This chapter outlines the main elements of good marketing planning, strategy and tactics, and demonstrates how these elements can be used efficiently and effectively in veterinary practices of all sizes. Throughout the chapter relevant frameworks and concepts are discussed in a practical and straightforward manner. The chapter also usefully compares the roles of sales and marketing in a veterinary practice, demonstrating how the two integrate. It also addresses the need for veterinarians to understand their different client groups, highlighting the value of segmentation analysis for building long-term 'competitive advantage'. Additional concepts such as branding and digital marketing are also introduced in the chapter. Finally, some valuable and cost-effective monitoring tools and techniques that can be adopted by veterinary practices to assess their marketing efforts are also discussed.

The branding theme is continued and further developed in chapter 8 by Cathy Coates. Reflecting the nature of the veterinary profession, the chapter focuses on developing a brand for a service rather than a product offering. The author notes that the use of branding to promote veterinary services is a relatively recent development, and that the potential benefits to be gained from the use of branding by veterinary practices and hospitals are not yet fully understood. In this chapter, students explore the three key dimensions of branding – brand identity, brand value and brand equity – and their application in the veterinary context. The author posits that the branding (or, in most cases, re-branding) process inevitably leads to a rethink of the overall values that the veterinary business represents and the image it wants to portray to its clients. Branding in the veterinary context essentially helps clients to better understand the value of the professional service being provided. Particular attention is paid to veterinary hospitals, with the author proposing a theoretical re-branding model that could usefully be applied.

Chapter 9, by Jeremy Phillipson, Amy Proctor, Philip Lowe and Andrew Donaldson, focuses on the important role played by the farm animal veterinarian as knowledge broker. As veterinary professionals, farm animal veterinarians are part of the knowledge-based economy in which they earn their livelihood by selling their expertise directly to clients. Indeed, they play a key role in enhancing the skills and development of tens of thousands of farming businesses. Thus they face complex and ever-changing calls on their expertise and are required to keep their knowledge up to date in practice. The chapter draws on recent research conducted by the Newcastle research team that explores the composition of field expertise and the role of field advisors in knowledge exchange. Essentially, 'field professionals' such as farm animal veterinary surgeons (but also agronomists, nutritionists, ecologists, etc.) act as intermediaries bringing science to the farm. Furthermore, veterinarians broker different types of knowledge apart from formal science; they also generate new knowledge and actively solve problems that they encounter as they strive to safeguard animal and public health. Veterinarians thereby build up their own experiential and experimental knowledge in and through practice. They are more than just transferors of knowledge from others; rather, they combine, translate and repackage information and draw on their own accumulated field knowledge to tailor it to the circumstances of the client. From an ethical perspective, this chapter also resonates with some of the concepts discussed in chapters 5 and 6 in relation to ethical business practice and veterinarians' requirement for vigilance as they go about their business of safeguarding animal welfare.

Part II of the book comprises a set of seven practical case studies, all contextualized within the broader veterinary business sector. Each case demonstrates a different veterinary/veterinary-related business scenario, and presents a particular business challenge for students to solve. This part of the book is supported by additional online case learning material, especially designed for busy 'mobile'-oriented students, and hosted by Elsevier's dedicated learning web platform.

The first case study, presented by Claire Denny, Sarah Baillie and James Gazzard in chapter 10, depicts the typical veterinary graduate taking her first steps in the world of work. Ellie Prior has been well prepared for the clinical demands she is likely to face but is less aware and certainly less confident of her role as an employee in a small enterprise. The case allows students to consider, through the eyes of a new entrant to the profession, the operations of a typical small animal veterinary practice. It explores the role of new graduates and their business interplay with more experienced colleagues and clients. Specifically, it focuses on the challenging topics of talking about money and charging for professional services in a clinical environment. This case study provides a mechanism which veterinary students, recent graduates, educators and employers can use to discuss a number of core veterinary business issues. The specific challenge for students in this case is to reflect on the business mistakes Ellie has made and help her avoid making them again in the future. When reading this case study, students might find it interesting to reflect on chapter 2, which discussed the various perceptions of the need for business skills.

In chapter 11, Izzy Warren Smith presents the case study of the Church Hill Equine Practice, which maps the successful start-up, survival and growth of a large-animal veterinary practice located in the Welsh–English borderlands. The case identifies the key factors that have precipitated and facilitated growth, from opportunity recognition to expansion, and traces the progression of Church Hill from a rural large-animal practice to a specialist equine clinic. Issues such as practice specialization, the profitability of a large-animal practice and the changing rural market for veterinary practice are addressed, along with an in-depth look at how Church Hill have developed good business practice by building on their areas of strength. The case highlights both the positive and negative aspects of practice management, from marketing through to staffing issues, and in so doing provides students with 'real-life' scenario-building frameworks from which they can not only apply entrepreneurship theory but also learn about the practicalities of running a rurally based veterinary enterprise.

The particular challenge for students is to draw on business and enterprise concepts to develop a growth plan to help move the business forward. In addressing this challenge, students might find it useful to reflect on some of the marketing concepts presented in chapters 7 and 8. In addition, students may find that the concept of the farm animal veterinarian as knowledge broker, as discussed in chapter 9, is particularly relevant here.

Cromlyn Vets is the case study presented by Colette Henry in chapter 12. In contrast to the previous chapter, this case focuses on a small mixed veterinary practice in Northern Ireland, established by husband and wife team Chris and Lynn Heffron. Practical veterinary business issues such as striving for and maintaining excellence in clinical veterinary care, maximizing resources, utilizing available expertise and retaining client numbers in the face of growing competition are discussed. The case provides students with an opportunity to really understand the challenges involved in developing and growing a small veterinary practice, and building up and sustaining the business over the long term. Essentially, Cromlyn Vets is a very successful and client-focused business, but the practice owners are very mindful of the changes taking place in both the wider and local veterinary marketplace. Students are challenged to apply marketing theories to propose an effective development strategy to ensure Cromlyn maintain their competitive edge in the face of new corporate competition. In this regard, students should find some of the concepts discussed in chapters 7 and 8 helpful.

De'Ath, Slaughter, Davis and Jones is the case study presented by Lynne Hill in chapter 13. This particular case centres on branding and discusses the process and decisions that need to be made by an old established practice that is about to relocate to new premises. The practice has grown from a farm-centric business to a small-animal one with substantial referral work. The study depicts the senior partner considering the changes that have occurred to the practice caseload over the years, and how the dynamics of the business have altered during that period. Examples of financial information for the business including the profit-and-loss accounts are illustrated for the reader to enable him or her to formulate an understanding of what is actually happening to the business. The challenge presented to the student is to determine whether it is now appropriate for the practice to engage in a total re-branding exercise and, if so, what form such re-branding should take. The case explores the processes required for a business to re-brand itself, and asks students to develop a strategy to fit the strategic direction that should now be followed. The concepts discussed in chapter 8 should be of particular relevance here.

In chapter 14, Cascade Veterinary Practice – the first of two case studies from Australian authors Adele Feakes and Diane Whatling – the impact of changing demographics is discussed. This is an interesting veterinary business case as it is based on a marital partnership. Strategy and planning for the Cascade Veterinary Practice has become less of a priority for the owners, with family responsibilities and personal issues taking priority, much to the detriment of the business. There are a number of problems in this business, and training and development of staff could be key to the future survival of the practice. Students are asked to consider all aspects of the business, including current financial key performance indicators, to work out a plan for the way forward. Essentially, a new business plan is required – one that is more in line with projected income analysis. This is quite a robust case, which will really challenge students. It relates to many of the concepts discussed in the theoretical chapters. Thus, while the marketing chapters will be invaluable here, students will also need to draw on some of the leadership theories discussed in chapters 2 and 3, as well as the management and ethics concepts from chapter 5, the latter being particularly relevant in the light of the alcohol issue articulated in the case.

Northington Veterinary Clinic, by Adele Feakes and Diane Whatling, is the focus of chapter 15. The veterinary clinic depicted in this Australian case study is tired and rundown, very much reflecting the state of mind of the principal veterinarian. Peter, Northington's owner, is contemplating retirement, and is considering making a succession plan. Jim, one of the veterinarians employed by the clinic, sees huge potential in renovating the practice. Currently, the organization is poorly structured, and staff morale is generally low. There is no clear strategic direction for the business, and the prevailing organizational culture is not very positive. A major reassessment of staff needs, including a training needs analysis and development plan, is imperative for success and must be actioned immediately. Financial accountability and cash flow are causing daily operational and legal issues due to poor management impacting on creditors. The current principal is also causing professional and ethical issues within the practice and with the veterinary surgeons board. Northington Veterinary Clinic requires a major makeover both externally and internally in order to retain current clients and attract a new clientele. The challenge here for students is to develop a plan that helps Jim determine whether taking over Northington and making the required renovations could actually give him a sufficient return on his investment. Once again, it will be useful for students to reflect on the concepts discussed in the leadership chapters.

The final case study, Parasol Kennels, presented in chapter 16 by Christopher Brown and Jane Taylor, focuses on the animal housing market. This case is different from the others as it was designed to help veterinary students explore innovation and sustainability within the broader veterinary and related sectors. It provides students with insights into the business development process with regard to both securing a market position and ensuring steady product innovation. The case shows how Parasol have managed to create competitive advantages around specific problems, developing solutions to meet the commercial and charity markets, and creating wider market opportunities for added-value products,

especially those relating to alternative energy solutions. Essentially, the case study highlights an entrepreneurial small business that has achieved a great deal since its inception. It also amplifies the challenges the business is facing in its bid to expand both within and beyond the UK market. Drawing on some of the marketing chapters in the book to articulate their proposals, students are asked to determine the most appropriate export opportunity for Parasol to exploit.

It is hoped that the diversity of perspectives included in this edited collection of chapters can offer valuable new insights into current veterinary business and enterprise curricula. The combination of theory and practice-derived contributions should help enhance understanding of veterinary business while at the same time encouraging students to draw on their latent creative and enterprise skills and abilities to solve some of the very 'real' challenges faced by veterinary business owners.

References

HEA – Higher Education Academy, 2005. Embedding employability in the curriculum: enhancing students' career planning skills. Report available at: http://www.heacademy.ac.uk

Henry, C., 2011. A critical review of contemporary practice in veterinary business education: report for the HEA BMAF network. November 2011. Available at: http://www.heacademy.ac.uk/hlst/resources/detail/resources/critical-reviews/business-education-in-veterinary-medicine

Henry, C., Treanor, L., 2010. Entrepreneurship education and veterinary medicine: enhancing employable skills. Journal of Education and Training 52 (8/9), 607–623.

Henry, C., Treanor, L., 2012. Exploring entrepreneurship education within veterinary medicine: can it be taught? International Journal of Small Business and Enterprise Development 19 (3), 484–499.

Jerving-Back, C., Back, E., 2007. Managing a Veterinary Practice, second ed. Elsevier, London.

Lowe, P., 2009. Unlocking Potential: A Report on Veterinary Expertise in Food Animal Production. Department for Environment and Food Rural. Affairs, London.

RCVS – Royal College of Veterinary Surgeons, 2006. RCVS essential competences required of the veterinary surgeon: day one competences. Available at www.rcvs.org.uk

Shilcock, M., Stutchfield, G., 2008. Veterinary Practice Management: A Practical Guide, second ed. Elsevier, London.

PART 1

Theoretical foundations

The need for business skills in veterinary education: perceptions versus evidence

Martin A. Cake   Susan M. Rhind   Sarah Baillie

CHAPTER OVERVIEW

This chapter presents a comprehensive review of both perceptions and evidence for the importance of business skills to the success of veterinary graduates. The veterinary literature yields ample evidence supporting the importance of business skills: notably, they are acutely perceived as a major deficiency in new graduates, and are positively correlated with successful graduate outcomes including income and employer satisfaction. However, in a paradox which perhaps reveals more about perceptions than reality, business skills are almost universally rated of relatively lower importance in surveys where Likert scale methodology is used.

LEARNING OUTCOMES

After reading this review chapter, students will be better placed to consider for themselves the following crucial questions:
- How important are business skills to the success of veterinary graduates? Why are they important, and what is the evidence for this?
- Do perceptions match reality, when considering the importance of veterinary business skills? If not, why not?

Introduction

Graduate attribute or competence frameworks are becoming increasingly important in veterinary education and accreditation. Several influential international bodies have introduced core competence standards into accreditation procedures. Notably, the Royal College of Veterinary Surgeons (RCVS, 2001) 'Day One Skills' and 'Year One Skills' framework (which has also been adopted by the European Association of Establishments for Veterinary Education (EAEVE) and the Australasian Veterinary Boards Council), and the recently released North American Veterinary Medical Education Consortium 'Roadmap' report (NAVMEC, 2011) include comprehensive yet distinctly different lists of core graduate-level competences. As in human medicine, there has been a recent shift towards the progressive inclusion of non-technical or professional competences – in the veterinary case, including business skills – in addition to the more traditional outcomes of discipline-based knowledge and technical skills. This trend creates the risk that expansive and unprioritized lists of 'essential' competences may contribute to curriculum overload, which is recognized as a major concern for contemporary veterinary education (Pritchard, 1989).

Despite the importance of these frameworks in guiding international veterinary education and curriculum design, the evidence to justify the inclusion of various competences has rarely been transparent. Very little work has been published to provide direct empirical evidence supporting the importance of various competences to graduate success, or even to document a clear consensus of expert opinion. Thus, while many veterinary competences may be intuitively *perceived* to be important, few are known to be associated with any tangible professional outcome related to graduate success. Lewis and Klausner (2003) used focus groups to identify six themes around a definition of veterinary professional success: personal fulfilment, helping others, balance, respect, personal challenge and growth, and 'meeting

© 2014, Elsevier Ltd.

a level of compensation that meets life needs and permits one to sustain growth in the profession'. Additionally, standard definitions of 'graduate attributes' would add employability and effectiveness of the university-to-workplace transition as indices of success at new graduate level.

The large, interrelated KPMG (Brown and Silverman, 1999) and Brakke (Cron *et al.*, 2000) studies are routinely cited as establishing 'a pressing need for business management to be included in veterinary education' (Lowe, 2010), though both are commissioned economic analyses of the broad state of the US veterinary profession, with little emphasis on graduate-relevant outcomes. Our aim in this study was to comprehensively review and synthesize all contemporary published evidence for the importance of business skills to the success of graduate veterinarians, in order to promote 'best-evidence' approaches to undergraduate veterinary education and curriculum design. An open definition of business skills was used, to encompass all aspects including practice management, financial acumen, and sensitivity to economic considerations and their communication. The theoretical approach used for the review was to 'triangulate' evidence from several potential sources: (i) *perceived* importance amongst stakeholders, derived from surveys or consensus-based processes; (ii) evidence of competence or deficiency in recent graduates, and its impact; and (iii) evidence correlating business competences with graduate-level outcomes associated with success.

Review methodology

The research question for our review was defined as: 'What evidence exists for the importance of business skills to the success of a veterinary graduate?' A systematic search was conducted of the published veterinary literature using a combination of electronic databases and ancestral search from cited references. Database searches included Scopus (SciVerse), Web of Science, Medline, CAB Abstracts, and Google Scholar, using the truncated term *veterinar** in combination with potential domain identifiers including *business*, *'practice management'*, *entrepreneur**, *economic**, *profit** or *income* (where * indicates wildcard character/s). Database searches were not time-limited, and grey literature was included where possible (e.g. by Google Scholar), to capture, for example, commissioned industry reports in the public domain. Potential sources were identified, reviewed and categorized on the basis of providing any of the following levels of evidence:

1. defined veterinary competence lists or frameworks, derived by a broadly consultative or expert, consensus-based method;
2. perceived importance, as surveyed within a stakeholder cohort (veterinary undergraduates, recent graduates, veterinarians, employers, clients);
3. perceptions of competence or deficiency in business skills of recent graduates; or
4. empirical or statistical evidence of an effect on (or correlation with) any graduate-level outcomes related to an unconstrained definition of 'success', including but not limited to employability, ease of transition-to-practice, patient outcomes, job satisfaction, or income.

Exclusion criteria included:

(i) papers detailing only opinion, without original research (these were examined for cited references only);

(ii) unpublished competence lists referencing a single institution (such as those maintained internally by many veterinary schools) or those formulated without a clearly articulated external or expert consultation process. However, surveys referencing a single institution's competence list were included, as this represents one standard study design;

(iii) papers outside of the veterinary discipline (this is acknowledged as a limitation of this review, as there may be translatable research from similar business-based health professions such as pharmacy).

Extracted data included the following: country of origin, study design and methodology (e.g. wording of survey question), sample size, business competence (s) referenced, and mean (or median, or modal, depending on study) rating or ranking for business skills. To allow comparison of different surveys of importance or competence, the relative rank of business skills was determined from relative rating or frequency count, relative to all surveyed competences (i.e. mixed knowledge, technical, and non-technical competences) or within non-technical competences only.

Review results

The primary database search yielded 4270 abstracts from 1951 to 2012; 234 articles were selected for further assessment and 45 were included as evidence in this review chapter. The most frequent sources were the *Journal of Veterinary Medical Education* and *Journal of the American Veterinary Medical Association*. The majority of the studies cited in this review chapter were conducted in the United States, though studies from the United Kingdom (7), Canada (4), Australia (5), and The Netherlands (2) also provided evidence.

Inclusion in competence frameworks

All published competence frameworks reviewed contained business skills, in most cases as a core domain (Table 2.1). However, there was considerable variation in the business competences described, ranging from novice level [e.g. 'elementary knowledge' (RCVS, 2001), 'introductory knowledge'

Table 2.1 Business competences included in consensus-based veterinary competence frameworks

Reference and source	Consensus process	Business competences
Pritchard (1989), USA	Draft developed by advisory panel of 10 distinguished veterinarians and educators, reviewed at workshop of over 200 invited delegates	Business and management skills including management of one's personal affairs
Walsh *et al.* (2001), USA	Draft developed by faculty then reviewed by advisory panel of 17 veterinarians including professional bodies	Introductory knowledge of veterinary business practice, which includes the following attributes: • A general understanding of the working environment of a typical veterinary practice, with an introductory level of knowledge of small business management and economics, including the economics of animal health and well-being and an understanding of the role of animals in agriculture
RCVS (2001), UK	Developed by expert working party, followed by modification after open consultation to the profession and professional bodies	• Be aware of the economic and emotional climate in which the veterinary surgeon operates, and respond appropriately to the influence of such pressures • Have an elementary knowledge of the organization and management of a veterinary practice, including: – awareness of how fees are calculated and invoices drawn up, and the importance of following the practice's systems for record keeping and bookkeeping, including computer records and case reports
Lloyd and Walsh (2002), USA	Structured workshop of 38 faculty and practice management consultants	The art and knowledge for a successful veterinary practice: • Business fundamentals • Marketing and promotion • Practice location • The fiscal enterprise • Managing human resources • How to evaluate a practice for sale • Why businesses fail
Collins and Taylor (2002), Australia/NZ	Workshop of 25 representatives of Australian/NZ veterinary faculty and professional bodies	An understanding of the business of veterinary practice: • Comprising business fundamentals, organizational systems, human resource management, Key Performance Indicators, and ongoing quality control • With due attention to health and safety, knowledge management, design of hospitals, and complaint management

Continued

Table 2.1 Business competences included in consensus-based veterinary competence frameworks—cont'd

Reference and source	Consensus process	Business competences
Lewis and Klausner (2003), USA	Focus groups at six sites, 281 veterinary professionals nominated by universities and veterinary associations	Business oriented: • Knows the goals of the organization and the dynamics underlying its success • Identifies and focuses on satisfying clients, constituents, or stakeholders • Builds or implements systems or processes that facilitate meeting organizational goals • Uses financial, management, or operational concepts to manage a project or organization • Fosters the best use of resources to meet organizational goals
Miller *et al.* (2004), USA	Structured workshops; five groups of 7–13 veterinarians representing production animal industry bodies	• (*Feedlot*) Demonstrate an understanding of overhead • Discuss the different taxes that affect the practice, the individual, and clients • Demonstrate an understanding of . . . client accounts, sales tax, interest, and depreciation • (*Cow/calf*) Evaluate the cost effectiveness of treatments • (*Swine*) Recognize the client as the customer
Bok *et al.* (2011), Netherlands	Focus group interviews with 54 recent graduates and clients, validated by Delphi procedure with 29 experts representing the profession	Entrepreneurship • Plan and organize one's own practice activities • Manage the pharmacy and product stock in accordance with quality standards • Efficiently contribute to business administration • Ensure a responsible and transparent system of quality assurance in one's professional work environment
NAVMEC (2011), USA	3 consultative meetings of approximately 400 stakeholders; reviewed by 9-member Board; feedback provided by 353 organizations and individuals	Management (self, team, system) • A working knowledge of business and financial concepts on a personal and professional level • An understanding of administrative and leadership roles

(Walsh *et al.*, 2001)] to practice owner/manager level [e.g. 'design of hospitals' (Collins and Taylor, 2002), 'practice location' (Lloyd and Walsh, 2002), 'leadership roles' (NAVMEC, 2011)]. There was also variation in the organizational unit described, with some referencing the individual practitioner [e.g. '. . . one's own practice activities' (Bok *et al.*, 2011), 'one's personal affairs' (Pritchard, 1989)] while others refer more to the practice unit. One common theme was sensitivity to fiscal or economic considerations. In the Pew Report (Pritchard, 1989), introduction to business management was listed as one of nine 'essential components of a veterinary education' (p. 149).

While competence lists were unranked, in the Delphi procedure followed by Bok *et al.* (2011) three of the four 'entrepreneurship' competences failed to achieve consensus in the first Delphi round (defined as >80% score as 'relevant' or 'very relevant') and were only accepted after discussion and revision.

Perceived importance

In surveys of the perceived importance of variously defined business skills (Table 2.2), business skills were almost universally ranked near the bottom compared to other surveyed competences, even when

Table 2.2 Rated importance of veterinary business skills and deduced rank

Reference	Source	Survey question (and survey method)	Sample size	Business skill	Rating descriptor[a]	Rank *All*	Rank *Non-tech*
Veterinary undergraduates							
Walsh *et al.* (2001)	US	Importance for graduates of veterinary degree programmes (5-point Likert)	68	Introductory knowledge of veterinary business practices	Very valuable – very essential	60/62	22/22
Kogan *et al.* (2004)	US	Importance in defining a successful veterinarian or veterinary student (7-point Likert)	428	Business management skills	[Important]	18/24	17/23
				Financial success	[Somewhat important]	23/24	22/23
Rhind *et al.* (2011)	UK	Importance 'for easing the transition ...' (5-point Likert)	161	Business acumen	Indifferent	40/42	36/38
				Knowledge of veterinary practice management	Indifferent	41/42	37/38
Schull *et al.* (2012)	Aust.	Importance for new graduate veterinarians (5-point Likert)	83	Knowledge of veterinary business principles	Somewhat important	–	44/47
				Basic knowledge of accounting	Somewhat important	–	47/47
Recent graduate							
Weigel *et al.* (1992)	US	Importance to the successful practice of clinical veterinary medicine (5-point Likert)	109	Financial planning	Not particularly – moderately important	9/10	4/5
				Hospital management	Not particularly – moderately important	8/10	3/5
Fitzpatrick and Mellor (2003)	UK	'How important has [this] been to you ...?' (5-point Likert)	391	Business management	Not very important	33/33	4/4
Rhind *et al.* (2011)	UK	Importance 'for easing the transition ...' (5-point Likert)	90	Business acumen	Indifferent	40/42	36/38
				Knowledge of veterinary practice management	Indifferent	41/42	37/38

Continued

Table 2.2 Rated importance of veterinary business skills and deduced rank—cont'd

Reference	Source	Survey question (and survey method)	Sample size	Business skill	Rating descriptor[a]	Rank All	Rank Non-tech
Veterinarians							
Weigel et al. (1992)	US	Importance to the successful practice of clinical veterinary medicine (5-point Likert)	38	Financial planning	Not particularly important – unimportant	7/10	4/5
				Hospital management	Useful – moderately important	8/10	3/5
Stone et al. (1992)	US	'Based on your own experience, how important is . . . formal training in . . .' (4-point Likert)	200	'. . . how to factor into your decision-making the cost implications of treatment'	Very important	8/16	6/11
Walsh et al. (2001)	US	Importance for graduates of veterinary degree programmes (5-point Likert)	49	Introductory knowledge of veterinary business practices	Very valuable – very essential	59/62	21/22
Bristol (2002)	US	Most important skills needed for success in veterinary practice (free response)	514	Practice management and personnel management skills	[8.1% of respondents]	3rd	2nd
Greenfield et al. (2004)	US	'List 10 most important skills . . . [for new graduates]' (ranked free response)	1328	Business skills	[14.1% of respondents]	13/38	3/17
Martin and Taunton (2006)	US	Importance to private veterinary practice (ranking)	415	Business management	–	–	3/10
Doucet and Vrins (2009)	Canada	Important for 'my current primary professional activity' (4-point Likert)	617	Manage financial resources	Agree – strongly agree	_[b]	_[b]
Mellanby et al. (2011)	UK	Importance in a veterinary surgeon (5-point Likert)	304	Clear about cost of treatment	Important	17/21	13/17
Schull et al. (2012)	Aust.	Importance for new graduate veterinarians (5-point Likert)	30	Knowledge of veterinary business principles	Very important – somewhat important	–	39/47
				Basic knowledge of accounting	Somewhat important	–	46/47

| Table 2.2 Rated importance of veterinary business skills and deduced rank—cont'd ||||||||
Reference	Source	Survey question (and survey method)	Sample size	Business skill	Rating descriptor[a]	Rank *All*	Rank *Non-tech*
Faculty							
Lane and Bogue (2010a)	US	Importance for veterinary graduates (7-point Likert)	186	Business skills	[Agree]	–	13/14
Clients							
Mellanby *et al.* (2011)	UK	Importance in a veterinary surgeon (5-point Likert)	407	Clear about cost of treatment	Important	17/21	13/17

[a]Descriptor of mean, modal, or median Likert scale rating [in square brackets, where estimated].
[b]Scale too coarse to determine rank.
Rated importance within studies surveying the importance of various veterinary competences and deduced rank (within all competences, and non-technical competences only), sorted by stakeholder cohort and year of publication. A lower rank order (i.e. higher numerator) indicates the stated skill was rated of relatively lesser importance than others surveyed.

compared only to other non-technical skills. Relative rankings were broadly similar across all surveyed cohorts, including undergraduates, recent graduates, veterinarians, academic faculty, and clients. However, the descriptors for the mean or median Likert scale result in most studies remained within the 'important' or 'agree' range. Business skills were not included in the competence lists of several similar surveys of perceived importance (Coleman et al., 2000, Heath et al., 1996a, 1996b; Hoppe and Trowald-Wigh, 2000). Survey results from the United Kingdom and United States appeared broadly similar. Several studies comparing surveyed cohorts found that veterinarians rated business importance lower than other groups; for example, Rhind et al. (2011) found recent graduates rated practice management of lower importance than final-year students, and Mellanby et al. (2011) found significantly fewer veterinarians than small-animal clients thought being 'clear about the cost of treatment' was very important. Similarly, Lane and Bogue (2010a) found that 164 DVM-qualified faculty rated business skills significantly lower in importance than 22 non-DVM faculty.

In an exception to this general pattern, the three surveys of veterinarians finding the highest rankings for business skills were also notable for their use of aggregated free response (Bristol, 2002; Greenfield et al., 2004) or allocation ranking (Martin and

Taunton, 2006) methodology, rather than Likert-scaled ratings against predefined competences. When Bristol (2002) asked 514 alumni for 'the most important skills needed for success in veterinary practice', the response category 'practice management and personnel management skills' was third most frequent, after communication skills and clinical skills. Similarly, Martin and Taunton (2006) found (using a points allocation-based ranking exercise by 415 veterinarians) that business management ranked third in importance, after communication skills and ethical reasoning, from a list of 10 non-technical competences, with no difference in ranking between practice owners or associates. Greenfield et al. (2004) found that 14.1% of veterinarians included proficiency in business management in their top ten most important skills for a new graduate. Lloyd and Larsen (2001) found consensus among practice management consultants and faculty that due to 'consolidating, competitive, and capacity trends', business skills would become more important in the foreseeable future.

Perceived competence and deficiency

Business skills were rated lowest (or close to lowest) in three studies surveying self- or employer-assessed competence of recent graduate veterinarians. Butler

(2003) found a significant difference between ratings of competence in 'job-related financial skills' by recent graduates and their employers, suggesting a difference in expected standards. Business competences were rated slightly higher in a recent Australian survey of graduating final-year students against the RCVS Day One competences (Schull et al., 2011). However, business skills were not assessed in several similar surveys of graduate competence (Gilling and Parkinson, 2009; Greenfield et al., 2004).

Conversely, business skills ranked very highly in several surveys of perceived deficiency of new graduates (Table 2.3). Walsh et al. (2002) found that knowledge of business practice was both the most frequently cited 'major deficiency' and the most frequent suggestion for additions to a proposed list of graduate expectations (111/235 responses). Jaarsma et al. (2008) asked 297 graduates to list topics they felt should have been covered on the basis of their experiences, and practice/business management was clearly the most frequent response (nearly half of the respondents). In qualitative surveys, Routly et al. (2002) identified financial skills as one of three 'particularly difficult' demands for the new graduate, reported as causing problems for 47% of respondents, particularly the appreciation of their own time and advice, and difficulties with appropriate estimates. Riggs et al. (2001) similarly found that 'gaining commercial awareness' was perceived as one of the most difficult aspects of work by 134 recent graduates, and was rated significantly more difficult by graduates compared to experienced veterinarians. Lewis and Klausner's (2003) focus groups also identified 'obtaining business and political acumen – understanding how business works and how business goals are translated into action' as one of six key 'environmental challenges' faced by veterinarians.

Coleman et al. (2000) asked 304 employers for specific issues of importance within various competence domains, and found the most cited issue within veterinarian–client communication was 'explaining cost to client'. When the same employers were asked to suggest competences required of graduates in the 21st century that were currently under-taught, the most cited response category was 'business management, including marketing and accountancy' (Coleman et al., 2000). The KPMG study (Brown and Silverman, 1999) found that in veterinarian focus groups 'many said that they did not get enough management, communications, and other skills necessary for non-private practice'. Similarly, 'many'

of the 34 senior partners surveyed by Routly et al. (2002) sought greater curriculum commitment to financial/legal issues. However, expected entry levels of proficiency may not necessarily be high; the 846 equine practitioners surveyed by Hubbell et al. (2008) indicated, on average, only the relatively modest expectation that new graduates should 'understand the cost of maintaining a veterinary practice' with 'much supervision'.

Graduate outcomes

Two clusters of evidence linked to graduate outcomes were identified in this review. Firstly, several related, widely cited US studies report an association between business acumen and income. The Brakke management and behaviour study (Cron et al., 2000) found that greater 'financial acumen' (measured as ability to define financial terms) was correlated with higher average incomes, and concluded that most veterinarians could increase their income through improved business practices. However, it should be noted that only practice owners were surveyed, with veterinary associates specifically excluded from this aspect of the study because it was thought they 'have no direct influence on the financial management of the practice'. Volk et al. (2005) also found business orientation and financial acumen, in this case measured by self-assessment questionnaires, to be strongly correlated with income. However, survey questions such as 'I feel confident about managing the financial concepts of my business' (a statement found to have one of the highest correlations with income) might also be interpreted as biased towards practice owners, and not transferable to new graduates.

Secondly, some published evidence links business skills to employability, in the sense of gaining employment and employer satisfaction. The KPMG report (Brown and Silverman, 1999) found in extensive surveys of veterinarians and veterinary employers that business skills were 'widely perceived by all [employer] groups as required skills to succeed in a traditional veterinary job', and also found evidence that increased veterinary training in financial and business skills may broaden employment opportunities by allowing veterinary graduates to 'better compete for veterinary related jobs for which a veterinary medical degree is not a prerequisite'. More recently, Danielson et al. (2012) used regression analysis to determine that employer-rated business skills of recent graduates (assessed by the paired test items 'perform

Table 2.3 Perceptions of graduates' competence or deficiency in business skills

Author(s)	Source	Survey cohort	Sample size	Business skill	Rating description	Rank All	Rank Non-tech
Perceived competence							
Tinga et al. (2001)	Canada	Recent graduates	142	Assisting clients with limited funds to make treatment decisions	[10% do not feel competent]	–	–
Butler (2003)	Canada	Employers	43	Job-related financial skills	Good [clinical proficiency of recent graduates]	40/41	17/17
		Recent graduate 7–10 months	125	Job-related financial skills	Very good	39/41	14/17
Hardin and Ainsworth (2007)	USA	Alumni	74	Introductory knowledge of veterinary business practices	[somewhat unprepared]	20/20	7/7
Jaarsma et al. (2008)	Netherlands	Recent graduate 24 months	134	Manage a practice/business	Disagree [that veterinary training sufficiently prepared me]	29/29	16/16
Schull et al. (2011)	Australia	Graduating final-year students	102	Aware of the economic and emotional climate in which the veterinarian operates …	Agree [that I am aware]	16/41	10/14
				Elementary knowledge of the organization and management of a veterinary practice … [including fees]	Agree [that I have elementary knowledge]	31/41	13/14
Perceived deficiency							
Weigel et al. (1992)	USA	Recent graduates	105	Financial planning	['areas in which new graduates are most deficient']	1/11	2/5
				Hospital management		1/11	1/5
		Employers	32	Financial planning		6/11	3/5
				Hospital management		4/11	2/5
Walsh et al. (2002)	USA	Alumni and employers	226	A general understanding of the working environment of a typical veterinary practice, with an introductory level of knowledge of small business management and economics …	Top-ranked 'major deficiency' – 15.9% of respondents	2/12	1/9

From surveys of self- and employer assessment, and deduced rank (within all competences, and non-technical competences only). For perceived competence, a lower rank order (i.e. higher numerator) indicates the stated skill was rated as relatively lower competence than others surveyed. For perceived deficiency, the higher the rank order (i.e. lower numerator), the more the stated business skill was thought to be deficient.

business-related tasks' and 'control expenses and maximize revenue') were one of only three non-technical skills subscales (along with interpersonal skills and problem-solving) to be positively correlated with overall employer satisfaction. Overall, non-technical skills accounted for 64% of the variance in employer satisfaction. However, in an Australian study of selection criteria used by employers (Heath and Mills, 2000), business skills were not surveyed, and only 9 of 126 employers responding to the invitation to list other attributes said they take into account 'an interest in business, sales and profit'.

Discussion

This review chapter cites a considerable body of evidence (summarized in Table 2.4), which – from any objective perspective – would normally amply justify the importance of any given competence as an educational priority: business skills are consistently included in competence frameworks defined by broadly consultative or expert consensus; they are acutely perceived as a deficiency in graduates, by both graduates and their employers; and they are linked to outcome measures associated with success, including income and employability. The quantity of the latter category of 'empirical', outcomes-linked evidence may seem modest, but in reality is much greater than equivalent evidence supporting many other competences accepted as 'essential'. However, these data must be reconciled with the contrary but consistent phenomenon that veterinarians and other stakeholders rate (by Likert scales) the *perceived* importance of business skills well below that of other listed skills. A further paradox exists in that several studies using a different survey methodology (free-response questions or ranking allocation) revealed a much higher perceived importance. Rhind *et al.* (2011) similarly found that while business acumen was rated poorly by Likert scale, qualitative data from focus groups simultaneously revealed a theme of understanding why it is important and should be rated higher. Unlike some previously observed shifts in 'flawed' undergraduate perceptions of veterinary competences (Heath *et al.*, 1996a), there is some evidence that the rated importance of business skills *decreases* across the transition to practice, and is lowest in graduate veterinarians (Rhind *et al.*, 2011) and veterinary faculty (Lane and Bogue, 2010a).

It should be acknowledged that a *comparatively* low rating does not necessarily imply that business skills are unimportant, though scrutiny of like-ranked competences provides a relative benchmark. For example, respondents in Walsh *et al.* (2001) rated business practices a mean of 3.38 on a 5-point Likert scale – thus between 'very valuable' and 'very essential' for graduates to have attained – yet they were ranked below 'normal growth patterns' and 'medical record keeping', and only above 'information technology', 'breed recognition', and 'non-traditional therapies', from a very comprehensive list of 62 surveyed competences.

One possible explanation for the relatively poor perception of business skills may be methodological

---

Table 2.4 Summary of evidence for and against the importance of business skills to the success of a veterinary graduate

Evidence FOR	Evidence AGAINST
• Business skills are included in all published, consensus-based veterinary competence frameworks • Business skills are cited as important skills in free-response or ranking surveys of veterinarians • Business skills are one of the weakest competences in new graduates, and this is perceived as a major deficiency by graduates and employers • Lack of confidence with financial aspects is a major difficulty for new graduates • Business orientation and financial acumen are correlated with success, defined as income • Business skills are correlated with employer satisfaction, and may broaden employment opportunities	• Business skills are typically rated of lower importance compared to other competences, when surveyed by Likert scale methodology

bias associated with Likert-scaled surveys, particularly the potential for 'evaluation apprehension' bias. This is respondent bias due to a subconscious feeling that the researcher is 'evaluating' their beliefs, and that some beliefs may be more acceptable than others. Coe *et al.* (2007) found a theme in veterinarian focus groups of a general unease about discussing the costs of veterinary care with clients, rooted in experiences of feeling guilty or undervalued. Similar feelings (of guilt for monetarily valuing their services) were voiced in the graduate surveys of Routly *et al.* (2002). There is strong evidence that veterinarians are not intrinsically motivated by money. Cron *et al.* (2000) found no significant correlation between mean income and job satisfaction, and Brown and Silverman (1999) found that veterinarians ranked income seventh on a list of eight reasons for choosing the profession, below the 'desire to work outdoors'. Rhind *et al.* (2011) found a qualitative theme in focus groups that students and graduates 'don't like to think of themselves as part of a business', and feel allegiance with ethical and welfare concerns where these are perceived as conflicting with economics. Together, this evidence suggests that veterinarians may feel, consciously or subconsciously, that business skills are a less noble or worthy aspect of practice, and therefore modestly acknowledge their importance without elevating them as a priority.

Although noting low competence in a skill does not of course automatically signal its importance, in this case competence data are clearly correlated with evidence from both rating and free-response surveys (Jaarsma *et al.*, 2008; Walsh *et al.*, 2002; Weigel *et al.*, 1992) that business skills are perceived as a key deficiency by graduates and their employers. This may indicate that business skills are under-taught (or perhaps 'under-learned'). The Lowe report, amongst others, reports clear evidence from working groups that 'insufficient attention is given in the selection, training and professional development of veterinarians to prepare them to run small businesses' (Lowe, 2010, p. 55). Qualitative focus group findings from the KPMG study (Brown and Silverman, 1999) suggest why this might be the case: 'many' participants said they were not taught enough practice management, yet 'all' agreed it would be difficult for schools to provide such skills due to curriculum overload, and 'many' felt it better to make these an admissions prerequisite. Lane and Bogue (2010b) surveyed faculty from US veterinary schools and found that only 56% agreed that it was their

responsibility to teach business skills, and this was probably related to equally low self-reported preparedness to teach them. In a survey of self-assessed communication and ethics competences, only 38% of faculty agreed with the statement, 'discussing payment and costs of care with clients is easy for me', and this item was also one of the lowest among undergraduates surveyed (Fogelberg and Farnsworth, 2009).

The paradox of acutely perceived deficiency but not importance may also be related to mismatch between graduate and employer expectations, as suggested by Butler's (2003) findings. For a new graduate, business aspects may be associated more with the 'lows' than the 'highs' of the job, in terms of steep expectations and critical feedback from both the client and employer. Thus business skills may be recognized as a major deficiency, because lack of business confidence regularly causes problems or frustration (Riggs *et al.*, 2001; Routly *et al.*, 2002), yet be denied as an important core quality of a veterinarian.

It is also possible that business skills are only valued once mastered, although the absence of higher ratings in veterinarian or employer cohorts (at least by Likert-scaled surveys) argues against this hypothesis. Deficiency in new graduates should, therefore, be interpreted in conjunction with findings such as those of Volk *et al.* (2005) that standard business practices are underutilized in US veterinary practices despite clear correlation with income, and that only 19% of veterinarians agree strongly with the statement, 'I feel confident about managing the financial concepts of my business'. Thus lack of business-related competences in graduates is symptomatic of a profession-wide deficiency, entirely consistent with the universally low ratings of importance reviewed here, while at the same time invalidating them. As the Lowe report (2010, p. 55) concluded, 'veterinarians' generally poor self-image of themselves as professional businessmen and women is both a cause and a consequence'.

Conclusions

This first comprehensive review of the topic summarizes evidence substantiating the importance of business skills to the success of graduate veterinarians. The poor perception of business skills among veterinary stakeholder groups continues to represent a special challenge for veterinary education, as articulated by Lowe (2010, p. 54): 'few [students are] motivated by the potential for a career in a business environment. This strikes me as a recipe not only for poor commercial performance but also for professional disillusionment . . . my impression of the veterinary profession is of scientific professionalism rather than a strong self-identity as providers of services to business. These aspirations are not incompatible and must be pursued jointly.' The consistency of this paradox suggests a deep-rooted psychological phenomenon that must be addressed and overcome in education. As a result of our review, we propose the following recommendations:

- Veterinary schools and accrediting bodies should clearly define an appropriate set of business competences important to support graduates' transition to practice. It is clear that the full range of competences defined in Table 2.1 is unachievable at new-graduate level, and dialogue must continue to agree which are essential graduate-level competences, and which are more appropriate to postgraduate-level training (Brown and Silverman, 1999; Lowe, 2010).

- It will likely be more fruitful to focus on modest and achievable competences than to expect new graduates to shoulder the burden to redress an endemic, profession-wide deficiency in business competence. Defined competences must be of clear and immediate relevance to recent graduates, noting Ilgen's (2002) conjecture that business skills are less valued because students intuitively perceive they will not be needed until much later in their career.

- As a minimum, effort should be made to clearly elaborate the importance of business skills as reviewed here; it should be assumed that most students will not intuitively see their relevance. Low perceptions of the importance of business skills should be recognized as the major barrier to veterinary business education, and attitudinal change should be viewed as the foremost educational objective. Attitudinal change in itself may be enough to influence graduate outcomes; for example, Henry and Treanor (2010) posit the flow-on effects of fostering an 'entrepreneurial mindset' on self-confidence and employability.

- More research should be conducted to support the typically cited US industry studies (Brown and Silverman, 1999; Cron et al., 2000; Volk et al., 2005), which are broad-based economic studies of the profession rather than entry-level outcomes.

Future studies should aim to substantiate the importance of business skills (and many other non-technical competences) by linking competence to authentic graduate outcomes, as demonstrated in the recent study of employer satisfaction by Danielson et al. (2012). Other potential outcome measures may include employability, ease of transition-to-practice, self-confidence, job satisfaction, and stress or happiness subscales.

Summary

This chapter has summarized the evidence substantiating the importance of business skills to the success of graduate veterinarians. It has also highlighted the poor perceptions of business skills among many stakeholder groups including students, graduates and employers. As a result of their review, the authors have offered a number of recommendations to help veterinary schools and educators deal with this issue.

Review questions

1. There are many ways of defining 'success' in the context of a veterinary graduate. Which aspects of success do you think might depend, directly or indirectly, on good business skills?
2. Examine the various veterinary business competences listed in Table 2.1. Do you think all of these are appropriate competences at new graduate level? Which do you think are most important?
3. One possible explanation for the comparatively low ratings of perceived importance of business skills is 'evaluation apprehension' bias, implying that business skills are felt to be less worthy than other competences. Do you agree with this assessment?
4. How important did you think business skills were before reading this chapter? Has the evidence summarized here changed your mind?

Acknowledgements

The authors wish to thank Hamish Macleod and Stephen May for their very useful advice on interpretation of survey data, and Marshall Dozier and Fiona Brown for their valuable assistance with the database searches.

References

Bok, H.G.J., Jaarsma, A.D., Teunissen, P.W., et al., 2011. Development and validation of a competency framework for veterinarians. J. Vet. Med. Educ. 38, 262–269.

Bristol, D.G., 2002. Using alumni research to assess a veterinary curriculum and alumni employment and reward patterns. J. Vet. Med. Educ. 29, 20–27.

Brown, J.P., Silverman, J.D., 1999. The current and future market for veterinarians and veterinary medical services in the United States. J. Am. Vet. Med. Assoc. 215, 161–183.

Butler, D.G., 2003. Employer and new graduate satisfaction with new graduate performance in the workplace within the first year following convocation from the Ontario Veterinary College. Can. Vet. J. 44, 380–391.

Coe, J.B., Adams, C.L., Bonnett, B.N., 2007. A focus group study of veterinarians' and pet owners' perceptions of the monetary aspects of veterinary care. J. Am. Vet. Med. Assoc. 231, 1510–1518.

Coleman, G.T., Salter, L.K., Thornton, J.R., 2000. What skills should veterinarians possess on graduation? Australian Veterinary Practitioner 30, 124–131.

Collins, G.H., Taylor, R.M., 2002. Attributes of Australasian veterinary graduates: report of a workshop held at the Veterinary Conference Centre, Faculty of Veterinary Science, University of Sidney, January 28–29, 2002. J. Vet. Med. Educ. 29, 71–72.

Cron, W.L., Slocum Jr., J.V., Goodnight, D.B., Volk, J.O., 2000. Executive summary of the Brakke management and behavior study. J. Am. Vet. Med. Assoc. 217, 332–338.

Danielson, J.A., Wu, T.F., Fales-Williams, A.J., et al., 2012. Predictors of employer satisfaction: technical and non-technical skills. J. Vet. Med. Educ. 39, 62–70.

Doucet, M.Y., Vrins, A., 2009. The importance of knowledge, skills, and attitude attributes for veterinarians in clinical and non-clinical fields of practice: a survey of licensed veterinarians in Quebec. Canada. J. Vet. Med. Educ. 36, 331–342.

Fitzpatrick, J.L., Mellor, D.J., 2003. Survey of the views of graduates (1993 to 1997) on the undergraduate veterinary clinical curriculum in the British Isles. Vet. Rec. 153, 393–396.

Fogelberg, K., Farnsworth, C.C., 2009. Faculty and students' self-assessment of client communication skills and professional ethics in three veterinary medical schools. J. Vet. Med. Educ. 36, 423–428.

Gilling, M.L., Parkinson, T.J., 2009. The transition from veterinary student to practitioner: a 'make or break' period. J. Vet. Med. Educ. 36, 209–215.

Greenfield, C.L., Johnson, A.L., Schaeffer, D.J., 2004. Frequency of use of various procedures, skills, and areas of knowledge among veterinarians in private small animal exclusive or predominant practice and proficiency expected of new veterinary school graduates. J. Am. Vet. Med. Assoc. 224, 1780–1787.

Hardin, L.E., Ainsworth, J.A., 2007. An alumni survey to assess self-reported career preparation attained at a US veterinary school. J. Vet. Med. Educ. 34, 683–688.

Heath, T.J., Mills, J.N., 2000. Criteria used by employers to select new graduate employees. Aust. Vet. J. 78, 312–316.

Heath, T.J., Lynch-Blosse, M., Lanyon, A., 1996a. A longitudinal study of veterinary students and recent graduates. 2. Views of the veterinary profession. Aust. Vet. J. 74, 297–300.

Heath, T.J., Lanyon, A., Lynch-Blosse, M., 1996b. A longitudinal study of veterinary students and recent graduates. 3. Perceptions of veterinary education. Aust. Vet. J. 74, 301–304.

Henry, C., Treanor, L., 2010. Entrepreneurship education and veterinary medicine: enhancing employable skills. Education and Training 52, 607–623.

Hoppe, A., Trowald-Wigh, G., 2000. Student versus faculty attitudes toward the veterinary medical profession and education. J. Vet. Med. Educ. 27, 17–23.

Hubbell, J.A.E., Saville, W.J.A., Moore, R.M., 2008. Frequency of activities and procedures performed in private equine practice and proficiency expected of new veterinary school graduates. J. Am. Vet. Med. Assoc. 232 (1), 42–46.

Ilgen, D.R., 2002. Skills, knowledge, aptitudes, and interests for veterinary practice management: fitting personal characteristics to situational demands. J. Vet. Med. Educ. 29, 153–156.

Jaarsma, D.A., Dolmans, D.H., Scherpbier, A.J., van Beukelen, P., 2008. Preparation for practice by veterinary school: a comparison of the perceptions of alumni from a traditional and an innovative veterinary curriculum. J. Vet. Med. Educ. 35, 431–438.

Kogan, L.R., McConnell, S.L., Schoenfeld-Tacher, R., 2004. Gender differences and the definition of success: male and female veterinary students' career and work performance expectations. J. Vet. Med. Educ. 31, 154–160.

Lane, I.F., Bogue, E.G., 2010a. Faculty perspectives regarding the importance and place of nontechnical competencies in veterinary medical education at five North American colleges of veterinary medicine. J. Am. Vet. Med. Assoc. 237, 53–64.

Lane, I.F., Bogue, E.G., 2010b. Perceptions of veterinary faculty members regarding their responsibility and preparation to teach non-technical competencies. J. Vet. Med. Educ. 37, 238–247.

Lewis, R.E., Klausner, J.S., 2003. Nontechnical competencies underlying career success as a veterinarian. J. Am. Vet. Med. Assoc. 222, 1690–1696.

Lloyd, J.W., Larsen, E.R., 2001. Veterinary practice management: teaching needs as viewed by consultants and teachers. J. Vet. Med. Educ. 28, 16–21.

Lloyd, J.W., Walsh, D.A., 2002. Template for a recommended curriculum in 'Veterinary Professional Development and Career Success'. J. Vet. Med. Educ. 29, 84–93.

Lowe, P., 2010. Unlocking Potential. A report on veterinary expertise in food animal production. Department of

Environment, Food and Rural Affairs, London.http://archive.defra.gov.uk/foodfarm/policy/animalhealth/vservices/pdf/lowe-vets090806.pdf.

Martin, F., Taunton, A., 2006. Perceived importance and integration of the human–animal bond in private veterinary practice. J. Am. Vet. Med. Assoc. 228, 522–527.

Mellanby, R.J., Rhind, S.M., Bell, C., et al., 2011. Perceptions of clients and veterinarians on what attributes constitute 'a good vet'. Vet. Rec. 168, 616.

Miller, R.B., Hardin, L.E., Cowart, R.P., Ellersieck, M.R., 2004. Practitioner-defined competencies required of new veterinary graduates in food animal practice. J. Vet. Med. Educ. 31, 347–365.

NAVMEC, 2011. Roadmap for Veterinary Medical Education in the 21st Century: Responsive, Collaborative, Flexible. North American Veterinary Medical Education Consortium, Washington.

Pritchard, W.R., 1989. Future directions for veterinary medicine. Pew National Veterinary Education Program, Durham.

RCVS, 2001. Veterinary Education and Training: A Framework for 2010 and Beyond. Royal College of Veterinary Surgeons, London A consultation paper prepared by the RCVS

Education Strategy Steering Group, July 2001.

Rhind, S.M., Baillie, S., Kinnison, T., et al., 2011. The transition into veterinary practice: opinions of recent graduates and final year students. BMC Med. Educ. 11, 64.

Riggs, E.A., Routly, J.E., Taylor, I.R., Dobson, H., 2001. Support needs of veterinary surgeons in the first few years of practice: a survey of recent and experienced graduates. Vet. Rec. 149, 743–745.

Routly, J.E., Taylor, I.R., Turner, R., et al., 2002. Support needs of veterinary surgeons during the first few years of practice: perceptions of recent graduates and senior partners. Vet. Rec. 150, 167–171.

Schull, D.N., Morton, J.M., Coleman, G.T., Mills, P.C., 2011. Veterinary students' perceptions of their Day-One abilities before and after final-year clinical practice-based training. J. Vet. Med. Educ. 38, 251–261.

Schull, D.N., Morton, J.M., Coleman, G.T., Mills, P.C., 2012. Final-year student and employer views of personal, interpersonal and professional attributes for new veterinary science graduates. Aust. Vet. J. 90, 100–104.

Stone, E.A., Shugars, D.A., Bader, J.D., O'Neil, E.H., 1992. Attitudes of

veterinarians toward emerging competencies for health care professions. J. Am. Vet. Med. Assoc. 201, 1849–1853.

Tinga, C.E., Adams, C.L., Bonnett, B.N., Ribble, C.S., 2001. Survey of veterinary technical and professional skills in students and recent graduates of a veterinary college. J. Am. Vet. Med. Assoc. 219, 924–931.

Volk, J.O., Felsted, K.E., Cummings, R.F., et al., 2005. Executive summary of the AVMA–Pfizer business practices study. J. Am. Vet. Med. Assoc. 226, 212–218.

Walsh, D.A., Osburn, B.I., Christopher, M.M., 2001. Defining the attributes expected of graduating veterinary medical students. J. Am. Vet. Med. Assoc. 219, 1358–1365.

Walsh, D.A., Osburn, B.I., Schumacher, R.L., 2002. Defining the attributes expected of graduating veterinary medical students, part 2: external evaluation and outcomes assessment. J. Vet. Med. Educ. 29, 36–42.

Weigel, J.P., Rohrbach, B.W., Monroe, A.C., Warner, S., 1992. Evaluation of undergraduate orthopaedic surgical training by survey of graduate and employer veterinarians. J. Vet. Med. Educ. 19, 2–5.

Clinical leadership and professionalism in veterinary practice

3

Liz Mossop

CHAPTER OVERVIEW

Veterinary surgeons need to consider the development of their professional skills, especially leadership skills. Veterinary practice teams can be complex, and require strong leadership skills in order to deliver effective clinical care. Clinical leadership is, therefore, an important concept for graduates to consider, especially when implementing the requirements of the RCVS regarding clinical governance. With this in mind, this chapter explores the concept of clinical leadership, and discusses the various skills and behaviours necessary to become an effective leader within the veterinary profession.

LEARNING OUTCOMES

After reading this chapter, students will be able to:
* Understand the nature of clinical leadership and its application to all stages of veterinary careers.
* Explain the difference between leadership and management.
* Describe the members of the veterinary practice team and discuss their different roles.
* Describe the components of clinical governance and understand their application in the veterinary context towards the attainment of quality in clinical care.

Introduction

Being a competent veterinary surgeon requires more than the ability to diagnose and treat animals. A broader set of skills is required by the new graduate vet, with professional skills becoming increasingly important as the profession evolves and responds to challenges created by changes to the economics of pet and farm animal ownership.

Many veterinary surgeons work in leadership roles, whether they are owners of a practice or employed in senior clinical positions, making leadership skills an important aspect of these professional skills. Effective leadership is an essential component of any attempt to motivate employees or implement change within a veterinary practice. Even the most junior assistant veterinary surgeon is a leader, to some extent, to their support team and clients, meaning new graduates must consider their ability to influence others. Leadership is required in many different workplace situations, and will be tested by emergencies requiring fast decision-making and direction. Veterinary leadership is specifically challenged by the dilemma of leading and managing a successful and caring team, while maintaining a profitable business.

Veterinary surgeons are also increasingly employed in leadership roles by corporate practices. This can create problems for the leader and team concerned, as not every individual has the attitudes and behaviours necessary to succeed in such situations. Attention needs to be paid to the development of these areas, which may not be a natural focus of professional postgraduate training.

The term 'professionalism' – the attitudes and behaviours necessary to be an effective member of a profession – is frequently discussed in the medical context but is becoming a more important topic for veterinary surgeons, as the profession considers its role in society. This is especially true when considering global public health, in which veterinary surgeons should play a prominent leadership role (Wagner

© 2014, Elsevier Ltd.

and Brown, 2002). Veterinary leaders need to demonstrate professionalism, and 'leadership' is often included as an element of professionalism. There is a clear overlap between these two concepts, meaning that the development of professional skills should also improve leadership abilities.

This chapter will examine the concept of clinical leadership, and discuss the members of the diverse team who may require leadership within a veterinary practice. The skills and behaviours necessary to become an effective leader and professional will be described and applied in the veterinary context, and methods of developing these often neglected areas will be outlined. Leadership will also be discussed in the context of clinical governance, both concepts being required for excellence in clinical care.

What is clinical leadership?

Leadership can be broken down into three simple components (Davidson *et al.*, 2006):

* identifying a goal or target;
* motivating other people to act;
* providing support and motivation to achieve mutually negotiated goals.

Importantly, clinical leaders maintain some form of clinical role, and work in a collaborative style with other health professions and non-clinical leaders to achieve improvements in clinical care (Edmonstone, 2009). Their focus is on the patient or service provided, rather than on the organization itself, which tends to be the role of healthcare managers; in the veterinary context, this is the practice manager. As Treasure (2001) is keen to point out, however, leadership can be mistaken for 'being in charge', particularly by medical consultants who may be in charge of a team, without considering that they are part of a service and care network. This could also be true in veterinary practice, where a leader is often the owner of the practice and seen to deliver orders rather than actually lead a multidisciplinary team effectively.

It must also be remembered that leaders are even better placed to exert power and influence, and so these abilities must be used carefully so that privileges are not abused (Anderson, 2011). The personal power of clinical leaders could be much greater than that of non-clinical leaders, because of their perceived credibility by fellow professionals (Edmonstone, 2009). Professionalism and leadership could, therefore, be

seen as intrinsic to each other; indeed, within the veterinary profession, there is more of a tendency to discuss the latter.

Leadership and management

It is important to consider the difference between leadership and management, particularly in veterinary practice where the two roles may overlap to a large extent. Three main scenarios exist:

1. A non-clinical manager is employed to oversee the day-to-day running of the practice and manage human resources. The practice manager in this situation is the employee of the individual who owns the practice, and varying amounts of autonomy are given, with the owner ultimately retaining the leadership role.

2. A veterinary surgeon (likely to be the practice owner) may manage the practice, and also have a clinical leadership role during client- and patient-facing activities.

3. In the corporate-owned practice, veterinary surgeons may lead and manage clinical activities but leave non-clinical management jobs to a central management team. Veterinary surgeons are more commonly becoming part of this central team, for example as regional operations managers within a corporate structure.

The differences between leadership and management are debated extensively in the literature, with some resistance to definitions which categorize them as distinct entities, often citing management as systems and process based, and forgetting that leaders also 'must ensure that systems, processes and resources are in place' (Long, 2011). It is certainly true that a badly managed practice may also suffer from poor leadership, and vice versa, but ultimately whichever role a veterinary surgeon adopts there will be similar skill sets, which need to be developed in order to influence a successful team approach to patient care. The small size of many veterinary teams means that individuals often take on different roles, many of which require leadership skills. There is some discussion around the ethical nature of leadership and management, with the implication that leadership is more ethical than *managership*, because of the tendency of the latter to be more 'dictatorial' in style (Ross, 1991). Whether or not this is true, it is worth considering that leadership may be a more realistic approach in the ethical mine-field that is the veterinary practice.

Table 3.1 illustrates the different characteristics required for management and leadership. Veterinary surgeons are likely to need to develop characteristics from both the management and leadership list as they perform a dual role in many situations.

Table 3.1 The different characteristics of management and leadership

Aspect	Management	Leadership
Style	Transactional	Transformational
Power base	Authoritarian	Charismatic
Perspective	Short-term	Long-term
Response	Reactive	Proactive
Environment	Stability	Change
Objectives	Managing workload	Leading people
Requirements	Subordinates	Followers
Motivates through	Offering incentives	Inspiration
Needs	Objectives	Vision
Administration	Plans detail	Sets direction
Decision-making	Makes decisions	Facilitates change
Desires	Results	Achievement/excellence
Risk management	Risk avoidance	Risk taking
Control	Makes rules	Breaks rules
Conflict management	Avoidance	Uses
Opportunism	Same direction	New direction
Outcomes	Takes credit	Gives credit
Blame management	Attributes blame	Takes blame
Concerned with	Being right	What is right
Motivation	Financial	Desire for excellence
Achievement	Meets targets	Finds new targets

Source: Long (2011, p. 4).

It is thought that clinical leaders are more likely to take evidence-based, reflective views on healthcare, and that this may be in conflict with the scientific–bureaucratic model promoted by non-clinical managers (Davies and Harrison, 2003). This can lead to ethical dilemmas for the practising veterinary surgeon, who is trying to balance clinical leadership skills aimed at improving patient care and animal welfare with the need to manage a practice and make a profit. Equally, there is potential for practice managers to come into conflict with veterinary surgeons employed as assistants who are more junior clinical leaders. These individuals will need to develop their leadership skill set in order to convince a more bureaucratic manager of their actions, which may be more patient centred than practice centred. Ultimately, it is the responsibility of both to ensure the culture of the practice is effective, and to develop a good working relationship allowing everyone to work as a cohesive team.

The complex nature of the veterinary team

The veterinary profession has undergone a considerable number of changes over the last two decades. The changing nature of animal ownership and farming practices has increased the numbers of specialized small, large and equine animal practices, and reduced the number of traditional mixed practices, which are usually run by one or more partners. Practices are now commonly owned by shareholders within a corporate management structure, and ownership by limited company is common even in the more traditional partner-led organizations. This has meant a readjustment in management and leadership of these practices. Practice managers are often now a part of this environment, along with numerous other professionals and paraprofessionals working along-side the veterinary surgeons (Figure 3.1). Some larger practices have embraced these changes fully and now employ professionals other than veterinary surgeons and nurses, with the aim of developing a wider scope for offering different services to clients and patients. Other practices have maintained a more traditional veterinary team, and communicate with other professionals contributing to patient care as and when required.

To an effective clinical leader, both types of team can be challenging. The veterinary surgeon may

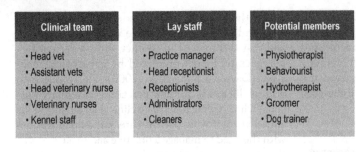

Figure 3.1 • An example of different team members in a small-animal practice.
Liz Mossop retains copyright to her original illustration.

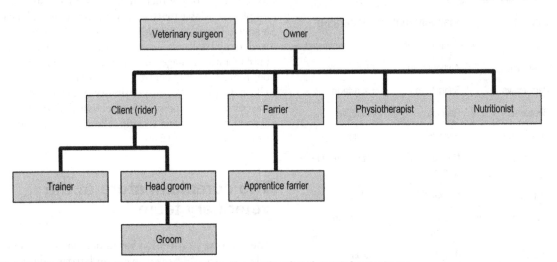

Figure 3.2 • An example of a complex team: the professional event horse team.
Liz Mossop retains copyright to her original illustration.

assume that everyone working in the team is aiming for the same ultimate outcome of excellence in patient care. However, tensions can develop when this is not the case, and communication and negotiation are of the utmost importance. The first step is to actually take on the responsibility of 'leader', which may not be a role every veterinary surgeon feels inclined to adopt, and some veterinarians may even leave leadership to the client. However, once the responsibility is identified, the second step is to decide how best to lead this complex team, and develop the skills and behaviours necessary to do so. This is required of even the most junior assistant. The different teams illustrated in Figure 3.1 must interact and communicate effectively. Leadership from veterinary surgeons is therefore essential.

In the situation illustrated in Figure 3.2, which depicts a more complex team, the vet may come under the direction of both owner and client, or these may be the same person. Leadership skills are very important if such a team is to function effectively, and the vet is ideally situated to lead this team.

Leadership styles

Social scientists, business theorists and psychologists have spent several decades studying effective leaders and their followers, and trying to establish the behaviours and skills necessary to develop a successful team. The classic leadership model first published in the 1950s (Tannenbaum and Schmidt, 1958), as shown in Figure 3.3, demonstrates a scale of influence during decision-making processes by leaders and their subordinates. This scale ranges from complete control by leaders through to total autonomy of subordinates. It is interesting to examine the behaviours described and consider leaders who feature prominently in the media. Politicians are a good example, but where on this scale do these leaders sit?

In reality of course, and as the authors of this model themselves came to recognize, leadership is more complex than the two roles of 'leader' and 'subordinate' may indicate. Leadership of teams requires a whole range of behaviours, and movement from one

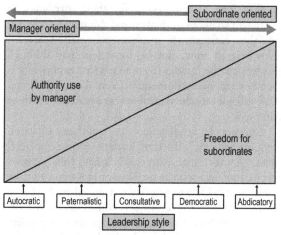

Figure 3.3 • The classic leadership model (Tannenbaum and Schmidt, 1958)

to another depending on context. Those being led also need to consider their behaviours in the context of the team in which they are working; leaders need to inspire this self-reflection and analysis.

The transactional leadership style

Transactional leaders tend to be more managerial in approach. They work with their team in a way that ensures members are goal orientated, with both parties achieving reward (Bass, 1990). Targets are defined and achievement incentivized, while deviation is corrected and may be punished. Transactional leaders can be both active and more passive in their approach to managing their subordinates by exception; they may look for deviation or intervene only when it occurs. Although this leadership style may be very effective in less complex organizations, it may be incapable of sustaining positive outcomes in multifarious and changing environments. Transactional leaders may fail to inspire the best performance from their team. This style of leadership is, however, commonly seen in veterinary practices, with employees working towards the right outcome for patients and clients, with or without extra financial incentives. There is an argument, therefore, that when trying to change procedures within a veterinary practice the transactional leadership style may be lacking what is required to produce the intended outcome. It has been demonstrated in the human hospital setting that an alternative leadership style, labelled transformational leadership, is

more effective in achieving better outcomes for patients and, interestingly, in achieving more effective cost control (Xirasagar *et al.*, 2005).

The transformational leadership style

Transformational leadership is visionary in its approach, inspiring followers to achieve through inclusive decision-making and empowering them to perform beyond expectations (Bass, 1990). As Edmonstone (2009) highlights, clinical leaders are more likely to achieve this through a collegiate, persuasive approach, based upon prior relationships of trust with their colleagues. This fits well with the ambitions of clinical governance and, in fact, a multifaceted, holistic leadership style may be the end result (Van Wart, 2003).

According to Bass and Avolio (1994), there are four key components ('four Is') of transformational leadership:

- Inspirational motivation
- Idealized influence
- Intellectual stimulation
- Individualized consideration.

With these 'four Is' in mind, a transformative leader motivates his or her followers by being an excellent role model, sharing goals and plans and having an optimistic outlook. Such leaders are innovative and keep looking for better solutions, even when an appropriate outcome seems to have been reached. For the veterinary surgeon, this means trust must be achieved with other members of the practice team and with their clients, who are essential components of a patient's healthcare team. Relationship building is crucial, including the use of empathy and rapport when carrying out consultations, as described in the Calgary–Cambridge consultation structure (Radford *et al.*, 2006).

Distributed leadership

This model of leadership moves away from considering the style of a single leader and instead considers multiple points of leadership within an organization. Leadership is considered as a social process, with spontaneous collaboration, intuitive working relations and institutionalized practice all being key elements (Gronn, 2002). The institution considers leadership to be every individual's responsibility to some extent, the idea being that this results in better collaboration and more cohesive teams.

This idea has definite application in the veterinary context, especially when considering the diversity of team members. Expertise from different sources can be combined to produce the best possible outcome for the patient. If effective collaboration and communication occur then the patient receives, for example, the best possible surgery, nursing care, postop care and rehabilitation. In the large-animal context, the herd or flock should reach maximum productivity while ensuring the best possible welfare standards. This is an interesting leadership evolution, and practices should consider whether it may be more effective to focus on systems that allow this to occur, rather than individual leadership skills (Swanwick, 2011).

Veterinary leadership skills

Leadership skills in healthcare are often discussed in the context of clinical governance (Hackett *et al.*, 1999). Reflecting on the changes to UK human healthcare delivery over the last generation (Breen, 2007), a similar situation can be seen in the veterinary setting; such changes, as outlined below, contribute to the need for clinical governance:

- movement from single-handed or small practices to corporate delivery;
- scientific and technological advances resulting in longer life and higher costs;
- government-funding strategies changing to include rationing and movement of some public health tasks to personnel other than veterinary surgeons, e.g. lay TB testers;
- better knowledge and access to knowledge by clients, so that outcomes are scrutinized and litigation is more likely.

The US medical literature is helpful when considering leadership in the veterinary context, as it includes cost control in its aims for clinical leaders (Berwick, 1994; Xirasagar *et al.*, 2005). This is a difficult component for clinical leaders to include in the UK context, where, perhaps wrongly, healthcare is not always viewed through an economic lens (Treasure, 2001). The US veterinary literature has tended to centre on leadership being required predominantly for economic reasons. Leadership skills are crucial for the growth of the profession, but often the essential skills of 'self-awareness, self-management, social awareness and relationship management' are lacking (Mase *et al.*, 2003). There

is therefore a requirement for these attributes to be taught to undergraduates, and this may be possible in the context of professional skill teaching. However, it must not be forgotten that although leaders can be 'made' to some extent, experience is another essential component (Van Wart, 2003) and this will not be gained until new graduates enter their first job.

Emotional intelligence is another oft-cited requirement of effective leaders and, as societal needs for veterinary surgeons change, this becomes even more necessary in order to produce emotionally intelligent leaders to respond to these changes (Lloyd *et al.*, 2005). As veterinary educational curricula begin to include the teaching of professional skills, there is the potential for leadership to become an inherent component.

However these skills are labelled within curricula, they are of increasing importance and will ultimately lead to improvements in the quality of patient care. The concept of clinical governance packages all these aspects into one, and so this will now be examined in more depth.

Potential conflicts between leadership and professionalism in veterinary businesses

Models of practice management have changed since the RCVS allowed non-veterinary surgeon ownership. Corporate groups have purchased large numbers of small practices, resulting in a structure of numerous small groups of veterinarians being managed by a mixture of clinical and non-clinical leaders. This has obvious potential to lead to conflicts between quality of care and economics – described by Edmonstone (2009) as a 'disconnected hierarchy'. This situation has been discussed extensively in the UK medical context, as doctors became increasingly uncomfortable and unhappy about the way they were being managed and the roles they were expected to fulfil within the NHS (Smith, 2001). Instilling leadership skills as part of professionalism teaching could help with this dilemma, encouraging professionals to develop their emotional intelligence and deal with uncertainty and change.

With the deregulation of tasks such as tuberculosis testing of cattle to allow other trained individuals to deliver them (Anon., 2005, 2011), vets also need to be ready to lead an interdisciplinary team at a practice level, continually striving to improve the quality of care, with financial success an added pressure and challenge to their professionalism. In order to do this, the concept of clinical governance will require discussion and implementation.

Leadership and clinical governance

A Government White Paper published in 1997 put clinical governance at the heart of the NHS as a method of improving clinical care (Department of Health, 1997). Defined as 'the framework through which organizations are accountable for continuously improving the quality of their services and safeguarding high standards of care by creating an environment in which excellence in healthcare will flourish' (Department of Health), the concept has been much discussed, with particular focus on the difficulties of changing a culture from one of 'blame' to one of 'continual improvement'. Instead of finding a scapegoat when errors and mistakes occur, governance encourages formal reviews of problems to examine the system rather than the individuals, where relevant.

Historically, clinical audit and governance have not been prominent topics in veterinary practice. However, this has recently changed with the release of the Royal College of Veterinary Surgeon's new Code of Professional Conduct (RCVS, 2012), which includes clinical governance as a required component of veterinary surgeons' actions. This topic will now become an essential element of veterinary professional behaviour, and effective clinical leadership will be crucial in order to implement the various different components.

The components of clinical governance are usually defined as education and training, clinical audit, clinical effectiveness, research and development, openness and risk management (Figure 3.4). Practices now need to consider these areas formally, and leaders must be trained effectively if changes are to occur successfully. It is recognized within medical organizations that none of these things can be implemented without effective leadership and culture change (Hackett *et al.*, 1999; Scally and Donaldson, 1998). If clinical governance is not being implemented within a practice employing a new graduate, this could present an opportunity for a junior assistant to develop and lead a governance team, with members drawn from all areas of the practice. Culture change may not be a realistic aim, but putting clinical governance

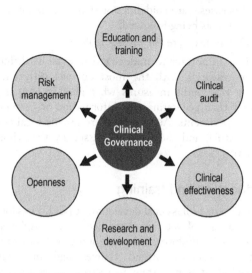

Figure 3.4 • The components of clinical governance

on the agenda of the practice is in itself a small change in culture, and could well result in positive cultural influences.

Components of clinical governance

Clinical audit

Audit has received some attention in the veterinary context (Viner, 2005), as it has been part of the RCVS Practice Standards Scheme and necessary to gain accreditation at Tier 2 and above. Clinical audit is a process of examining the quality of service and care offered systematically and critically, to measure whether expectations are being met. It is a cyclical process including the following steps:

- planning and selecting a topic;
- defining best practice and the standard at which something is to be measured;
- defining how the measurement will be done;
- collecting the data;
- analysing the outcomes;
- implementing change as necessary.

The entire cycle should then begin again with these changes in place. Deciding what should be changed at the end of the process can be difficult, and can be divided into three areas:

- Structures – does the practice have the correct equipment and staffing to achieve these standards; are staff correctly trained?

- Processes – are guidelines or standard operating protocols being followed?
- Outcomes – are the targets realistic?

It is important to understand how audit differs from research, with the most obvious difference being that audit measures what already happens, rather than generating new information or carrying out experiments. Audit results are usually local and contextual, and should be discussed by the whole practice team.

Education and training

Continuing professional development (CPD) has long been a part of veterinary practice. Most employers offer their employees a budget and give them time off in order to attend courses and meetings. However, it is important to recognize that training must go further than this and actually result in learning, and this can often be overlooked. CPD courses are expensive, and have a tendency to focus on clinical aspects of the job, at least for veterinary surgeons. Practices must consider requiring attendees to demonstrate their learning to other members of their team following CPD, and training should be broader than simply clinical updates. This is already happening in many corporate-led practices, which recognize the need for this and often implement a company-wide training policy. Leadership skills should also be developed in this way, and not just expected to be inherent components of individuals.

Clinical effectiveness

The quality of care provided to patients forms an important component of governance. While this is often measured during an audit cycle, it usually focuses on a single small aspect of care; governance requires a practice to monitor clinical effectiveness continuously and strive for the best possible outcome. If care is average, more untoward incidents are likely to occur, and this does not create a pleasant environment for staff or patients. The raising of standards and effectiveness from average to excellent is not easy, but ultimately should lead to better outcomes for employees, patients and practice owners. Evidence-based medicine should form a cornerstone of clinical effectiveness, despite the difficulties of this concept in veterinary medicine. Effective clinical leadership is vital to try to improve standards, and leading by example is a good way to influence those working with you.

Research and development

Research into new treatments and the development of new techniques may not be an inherent component of many veterinary practices on a day-to-day basis. However, research and development are important components of clinical governance because, ultimately, without them standards will not continue to improve. Practices should therefore welcome opportunities to take part in properly run trials, ensuring ethical standards are met at all times. These trials could range from collecting data retrospectively for epidemiological studies, which are essential to identify problematic issues and raise animal welfare standards, to much more complex trials. Veterinary clinical leaders should strive to be involved in such research and development opportunities.

Openness

Governance will become an ineffective process if clinicians are unwilling to divulge their practices and be open about errors and mistakes. This requires a real change in culture, and can only be achieved if clinical leaders demonstrate their own limitations and issues. An openness strategy within a practice may include an incident-reporting scheme and regular mortality and morbidity meetings. Critical incidents should also be discussed in an open forum, where individuals can express their opinions without the fear of blame. This process has become an essential component in, for example, aviation safety, as well as healthcare. Without a national reporting scheme (other than the VMD's adverse drug reactions scheme), veterinary practices are, in some respects, behind other industries. This is, perhaps, not surprising, considering the small business structure of the industry. However, while corporate ownership may change this, individual practices are perfectly able to implement their own culture of openness and discussion.

Risk management

The management of risk should be considered every day in a veterinary practice in order to work safely and effectively. Clinical risk is a straightforward concept to understand, but risk management should also include wider aspects of practice management so that it is viewed more holistically and includes environmental and operational risk as well as clinical aspects. Importantly for veterinary practices, financial risk should also be included. Risk management has obvious overlaps with the concept of clinical effectiveness because the reduction of risk should ensure better outcomes for patients.

Leadership development in the veterinary profession

Although specific leadership training has been delivered to early career doctors (O'Sullivan and McKimm, 2011), this rarely occurs in veterinary training. Individual components may be delivered to undergraduates in the context of professional skills, but there is a requirement for some kind of leadership development framework so that this skill set can continue to develop post graduation. Large practices or corporate groups may be able to implement a training framework across their clinical leaders as part of their continuing professional development. This has occurred extremely effectively in the US medical group Kaiser-Permanente, which has an extensive leadership development programme for doctors from their initial employment through to doctors working at senior management levels (Ham, 2008). Veterinary surgeons working in smaller practices, which are unlikely to use any kind of development framework, should not be deterred from considering their own skills. They can also be developed in a self-directed fashion, with individuals considering which skills they require and developing them reflectively using peer feedback. Some typical skills to consider are listed in Box 3.1.

A useful framework on which to base this development is the NHS Medical Leadership Competency Framework, in which five domains are highlighted (Box 3.2). These domains are expected to carry emphasis according to career stage – for example, a student doctor would focus on developing the personal qualities listed, while a senior consultant will be able to implement areas within setting direction. However, a student doctor is expected to understand the theoretical underpinnings of all sections, preparing them to work within the NHS as an effective team member.

There is definite application of this framework in the veterinary context. Practices deciding to embrace the concept of clinical governance will find that a framework like this gives their clinical leaders direction and reward for enhancing the skill set necessary to succeed. Veterinary schools should ensure that the

Box 3.1

Non-technical competences expected of effective veterinary leaders

Personal abilities
- Inner strength, multitasking, calmness, resilience, self-accountability

Personal characteristics
- Self-assessment, self-confidence, self-discipline, inquisitive nature, creativity, honesty and integrity

Interpersonal skills
- Empathy, listening skills, confidence giving, motivational

Change leadership and management

Visionary nature

Management skills

Leading, understanding and working in organizations

Source: Adapted from Lloyd *et al.* (2005).

Box 3.2

NHS medical leadership competency framework

1. Personal qualities
   a. Self-awareness
   b. Self-management
   c. Self-development
   d. Acting with integrity
2. Working with others
   a. Developing networks
   b. Building and maintaining relationships
   c. Encouraging contributions
   d. Working within teams
3. Managing services
   a. Planning
   b. Managing resources
   c. Managing people
   d. Managing performance
4. Improving services
   a. Ensuring patient safety
   b. Critically evaluating
   c. Encouraging innovation
   d. Facilitating transformation
5. Setting direction
   a. Identifying the contexts for change
   b. Applying knowledge and evidence
   c. Making decisions
   d. Evaluating impact

Source: Adapted from Academy of Medical Royal Colleges and NHS, Institute for Innovation and Improvement (2008).

personal qualities required of effective clinical leaders are developed within the curriculum, and underpinning theory relating to the other competences is also taught to undergraduates. In so doing, effective veterinary clinical leaders should be developed.

Conclusions

The challenges of leading a changing profession or veterinary practice are considerable, but effective clinical leadership should help ease the process. Effective leaders need to be developed, and their interactions with practice managers need to be considered. The implementation of clinical governance has become a priority for all practices and veterinary surgeons, and leaders will therefore need to develop and refine their own skill sets in order to execute these concepts effectively. Areas for improvement should be identified and measured against an expected standard; changes should then be implemented as required. Although some training will begin at veterinary school, many clinical veterinary leaders will have to develop their own skill sets. Practices should therefore consider leadership development frameworks in order to encourage practitioners to lead clinical teams effectively. Indeed, there is huge potential for larger practices or groups to implement a leadership development scheme, and this should be welcomed by the profession. Thus, while leadership training may begin at undergraduate level, it needs to continue throughout a veterinary professional's career.

Summary

This chapter has discussed the concept of leadership, relating it to the professionalism of veterinary surgeons working in practice. It has defined the different styles and models of leadership which may be demonstrated by veterinary leaders. The important concept of clinical governance, now required by the RCVS Code of Professional Conduct, has been described with a focus on the leadership skills required to implement these ideas. Leadership skill development was also discussed, with relevant frameworks and skill sets outlined.

Review questions

1. What are the components of clinical governance? Describe each one in turn and consider how these could be implemented in veterinary practice.
2. What are the key differences between leadership and management?
3. Consider your own leadership style. Can you identify where you may be perceived on the scale demonstrated in Figure 3.3 by your colleagues in practice?
4. Describe the transformational leadership style. What are the 'four Is' of transformational leadership?
5. What are the main challenges of clinical leadership within veterinary practices?

References

Academy of Medical Royal Colleges and NHS, 2008. Medical Leadership Competency Framework. Institute for Innovation and Improvement. Available at: http://www. leadershipacademy.nhs.uk/

Anderson, S., 2011. Leading organisations. In: Swanwick, T., McKimm, J. (Eds.), ABC of Clinical Leadership. Wiley-Blackwell, Oxford, pp. 24–29.

Anon, 2005. Pilot lay TB testing programme announced. Vet. Rec. 157 (5), 126.

Anon, 2011. RCVS Council members express concern about rise in lay TB testing. Vet. Rec. 168 (24), 630–633.

Bass, B.M., 1990. From transactional to transformational leadership: learning to share the vision. Organ. Dyn. 18 (3), 19–31.

Bass, B.M., Avolio, B., 1994. Improving Organisational Effectiveness through Transformational Leadership. Sage, Thousand Oaks, NJ.

Berwick, D., 1994. Eleven worthy aims of clinical leadership of health system reform. J. Am. Med. Assoc. 272, 797–802.

Breen, K.J., 2007. Medical professionalism: is it really under threat? Med. J. Aust. 186 (11), 596.

Davidson, P.M., Elliott, D., Daly, J., 2006. Clinical leadership in contemporary clinical practice: implications for nursing in Australia. J. Nurs. Manag. 14 (3), 180–187.

Davies, H.T.O., Harrison, S., 2003. Trends in doctor–manager relationships. Br. Med. J. 326, 646–649.

Department of Health, 1997. White Paper: The New NHS: Modern. Dependable, Stationery Office, London.

Edmonstone, J., 2009. Clinical leadership: the elephant in the room. Int. J. Health Plann. Manage. 24 (4), 290–305.

Gronn, P., 2002. Distributed leadership as a unit of analysis. Leadership Quarterly 13 (4), 423–451.

Hackett, M., Lilford, R., Jordan, J., 1999. Clinical governance: culture, leadership and power – the key to changing attitudes and behaviours in trusts. Int. J. Health Care. Qual. Assur. 12 (3), 98–104.

Ham, C., 2008. Doctors in leadership: learning from international experience. International Journal of Clinical Leadership 16 (1), 11–16.

Lloyd, J.W., King, L.J., Mase, C.A., Harris, D., 2005. Future needs and recommendations for leadership in veterinary medicine. J. Am. Vet. Med. Assoc. 226 (7), 1060–1067.

Long, A., 2011. Leadership and management. In: Swanwick, T., McKimm, J. (Eds.), ABC of Clinical Leadership. Wiley-Blackwell, Chichester, pp. 4–7.

Mase, C.A., Lloyd, J.W., King, L.J., 2003. Initial study results on future needs for leadership in veterinary medicine. J. Am. Vet. Med. Assoc. 222 (11), 1516–1517.

O'Sullivan, H., McKimm, J., 2011. Medical leadership and the medical student. Br. J. Hosp. Med. 72 (6), 283–286.

Radford, A., Stockley, P., Silverman, J., et al., 2006. Development, teaching, and evaluation of a consultation structure model for use in veterinary education. J. Vet. Med. Educ. 33 (1), 38–44.

RCVS, 2012. Code of Professional Conduct. RCVS, London.

Ross, J.C., 1991. Leadership for the Twenty-First Century. Praeger, Westport, CT.

Scally, G., Donaldson, L.J., 1998. Clinical governance and the drive for quality improvement in the new NHS in England. Br. Med. J. 317 (7150), 61–65.

Smith, R., 2001. Why are doctors so unhappy? BMJ 322 (7294), 1073.

Swanwick, T., 2011. Leadership theories and concepts. In: Swanwick, T., McKimm, J. (Eds.), ABC of Clinical Leadership. Wiley-Blackwell, Oxford, pp. 8–13.

Tannenbaum, R., Schmidt, W., 1958. How to choose a leadership pattern: should a leader be democratic or autocratic or something in between? Harv. Bus. Rev. 35, 95–101.

Treasure, T., 2001. Redefining leadership in health care. Br. Med. J. 323 (7324), 1263.

Van Wart, M., 2003. Public-sector leadership theory: an assessment. Public Adm. Rev. 63, 214–228.

Viner, B., 2005. Clinical audit in veterinary practice: the story so far. In Pract. 27 (4), 215–218.

Wagner, G.G., Brown, C.C., 2002. Global veterinary leadership. Vet. Clin. North Am. Food Anim. Pract. 18 (3), 389–399.

Xirasagar, S., Samuels, M.E., Stoskopf, C.H., 2005. Physician leadership styles and effectiveness: an empirical study. Med. Care Res. Rev. 62 (6), 720–740.

Leadership and management in veterinary practice

4

Brian Faulkner

CHAPTER OVERVIEW

Leadership and management are valuable commodities in any organization, and are crucial components of organizational success. This is also true in veterinary organizations because as an organization grows in size it requires a broadening range of professional skills and expertise, such as leadership, in order to remain effective. The aim of this chapter is to distinguish between the concepts of management and leadership, and to provide the reader with insights into the various leadership styles discussed in extant literatures. Leadership is investigated at various different levels ranging from its more externally observable or 'tangible' dimensions, as described in the traits, skills and styles approaches, to the more intangible or psychological dimensions, as described in the transformational and cultural models.

LEARNING OUTCOMES

After reading this chapter, students will be able to:
- Recognize the difference between management and leadership.
- Discuss the various models used to conceptualize leadership.
- Understand what leaders do and how they think.
- Appreciate how leadership relates to working in veterinary practice.

Introduction

Traditionally, veterinary practices have been established when a vet 'puts up their plate' and opens for business. In this model of veterinary practice the business founder acts as the main 'operator' or deliverer of professional services in the early stage of the business's development. At this stage of the business's life cycle, the need for sophisticated business and people management is less crucial. However, as the practice grows and the demand for its services increases, the business founder is faced with a choice, which creates challenges as well as potential benefits. The sole-charge veterinary surgeon has to choose whether to stay as a sole-charge vet or to take on new members of staff including more veterinary surgeons, veterinary nurses or receptionists. If the business founder decides to recruit additional staff in order to grow the business, he or she must know how to manage the spectrum of personalities, competences and agendas that inevitably accompany this transition. In other words, the business founder must now act as a leader and thus deal with the core challenge of leadership; how does he or she get the members of the team to work effectively together in pursuit of a common goal? Of course many, if not most, leaders and managers work within organizations and teams, which they themselves did not create. However, the challenge they face is exactly the same.

This chapter aims to explore some of the theories and models that have been used to explain the characteristics and strategies that leaders apply to meet the leadership challenge. The chapter explores how each theory relates to veterinary organizations ranging from the sole vet entrepreneurial set-up to the multi-site corporate chain. This, however, is not a straightforward task. While the literature on leadership in general is relatively broad, the literature specifically relating to veterinary leadership is virtually non-existent. In order to circumnavigate this

© 2014, Elsevier Ltd.

problem, the key models of leadership and people management will be described, followed by the author's own interpretation of how such models can be applied in the veterinary context.

Operators, managers and leaders

It is important to begin by recognizing the different perspectives, orientations and skill sets of operators, managers and leaders (Bennis and Naus, 1985; Kotter, 1990 Rost, 1991). Operators can be defined as the people who carry out the actual production or delivery of a business's services. In veterinary practice, these are the vets that perform the consultations and surgical operations as well as the nurses and the receptionists who support them. A manager is the person who supervises and assists the operators. Managers are focused on the efficiency and accuracy with which certain outcomes are achieved by the people and the systems that deliver them. There are many potential outcomes that can be measured in veterinary practice; these include clinical outcomes (e.g. number of postoperative wound infections), commercial outcomes (turnover, profit, number of transactions), client outcomes (satisfaction scores and willingness to recommend the practice) and staff outcomes (morale, ability to perform certain tasks). Each of these outcomes is called a key performance indicator (KPI). While some KPIs are commonly used to measure performance within the veterinary profession, such as commercial outcomes, there is no absolute list of KPIs which all veterinary organizations adopt to track their progress. Indeed, in the author's experience, a manager can make an immediate impact within their veterinary organization by simply identifying and defining which KPIs they wish to measure, and then making efforts to improve them.

It is, of course, possible for the same individual to act both as an operator and a manager, and this is very common in the traditional owner-operator model of veterinary practice. It is increasingly common, however, for individuals to act only as 'professional' managers within the veterinary profession, fulfilling roles such as practice managers or middle and senior managers within larger corporate groups. Professional managers such as these are drawn from a range of occupational backgrounds. Some originate within the veterinary industry, such as veterinary nurses and receptionists as well as veterinary surgeons, while others come from a non-veterinary background. This variety of backgrounds is often reflected in the KPIs, which different managers use to track the success of the veterinary businesses they manage. It is reasonable to suggest that the most effective managers within the industry will be those who use a range of KPIs to monitor the systems, which are critical to achieving a range of effective outcomes within the profession, i.e. clinical outcomes, client outcomes, financial outcomes and staff outcomes. The specific combination of KPIs that a manager uses is often referred to as their 'dashboard'.

Theories on leadership

Acting as a leader is distinct from acting as an operator or a manager, even though the same person can perform all three functions at different times. Leadership is often spoken of as if it were simply advanced 'management'. The presumption is that whatever the manager can do, the leader does more of and does it better. To equate management with leadership is to miss an essential difference between these two modes of working; it is like saying that vets are just more qualified nurses, when in fact they have different roles with different orientations and focus. Capturing the essence of that difference has been the subject of much research and debate, resulting in many different conceptualizations within the literature about what leadership actually is. The aim of the discussion below is to highlight the key features of each of these theories, particularly in relation to how they help us meet the leadership challenge, i.e. getting members of the group to work effectively together in order to achieve a common goal.

The 'Great Man' approach

Up until the latter part of the twentieth century, leadership was thought of as a primarily male, military and Western concept. The Great Man approach is based on the belief that leaders are exceptional people, born with innate qualities, destined to lead. Their followers' 'undisputed' deference to their superior status and innate brilliance entitles them to command members of the group to carry out their instructions without question in order to achieve their goals.

The trait approach

Traits are defined as habitual patterns of behaviour, thought and emotion (Kassin, 2003). This approach to understanding leadership evolved from the Great Man approach as a way of defining and identifying the personal characteristics which enable leaders to get people to work effectively together towards a common goal (Bass, 1990; Jago, 1982). Various researchers have identified a range of traits, and some of these are summarized in Table 4.1. Within the veterinary literature some authors have listed traits which they assert are critical to leadership and management within the veterinary context (Little, 2011; Sheridan and McCafferty, 1993); these are also included in Table 4.1.

The trait approach is intuitively appealing as it is tempting to conceptualize leaders as possessing specific talents that enable them to take charge and motivate themselves and others to do extraordinary things. This model is applied by identifying, recruiting and installing people with the 'right' traits into positions of command. This approach was common in the military. However, the weakness with the trait approach lies in the weakness of trait theories as a model for understanding and predicting how people behave in general (for a review see, for example, Dweck, 2000). Traditionally, trait models described people's behaviour without explaining how those patterns of behaviour develop in the first place or how they might change (Costa and McCrae, 1994; Goldberg, 1990; McCrae and John, 1992). Many trait theorists assume our traits are rooted in our biology and, as such, they assert that we cannot change very much (Costa and McCrae, 1994; Eysenck, 1982; Loehlin, 1992). Trait theories of leadership therefore assume you either possess the right traits for the job or you do not. Traits are assessed using self-report psychometric questionnaires whereby participants 'identify' their own patterns of behaviour, thought and emotion by rating themselves against the questions asked. Self-report questionnaires have been criticized, however, as a very inaccurate method of identifying an individual's actual talents. Similarly, trying to determine another person's traits over a short period of time (such as during an interview) has also proven to be inaccurate. Furthermore, it has been known for some time that

Table 4.1 Studies of leadership traits and characteristics

Leadership traits (non-veterinary literature)				Leadership traits (veterinary literature)	
Stogdill (1974)	Lord *et al.* (1986)	Kirkpatrick and Locke (1991)	Zaccaro *et al.* (2004)	Sheridan and McCafferty (1993)	Little (2011)
Achievement	Intelligence	Drive	Cognition	Good judgement	Vision
Persistence	Masculinity	Motivation	Extroversion	Entrepreneurial flair	Toughness
Insight	Dominance	Integrity	Conscientiousness	Psychological stamina	Fairness
Initiative		Confidence	Emotional stability	Decisiveness	Adaptability
Self-confidence		Cognitive ability	Openness	Delegation	Integrity
Responsibility		Task acknowledgement	Agreeableness	Whim resistance	Warmth
Cooperativeness			Motivation	Dependability	
Tolerance			Social intelligence	Application	
Influence			Emotional intelligence		
			Problem solving		

Source: Adapted with permission from Northouse, PG. Leadership: Theory and Practice, 5th ed. Thousand Oaks, CA: Sage Publications; 2010

the presence or absence of many of the key traits listed in Table 4.1 does not predict how effective a person will be as a leader across a range of situations (Stogdill, 1948). Few veterinary organizations within the UK currently use formal psychometric profiling techniques to identify and recruit staff in general, and leaders in particular. This has led to a lack of empirical data with respect to determining the usefulness of traits as a model for leadership within the profession. However, in the author's experience, most veterinary employers rely heavily on their own evaluation of a colleague's 'attitudes and traits' when they are deciding whether someone is suitable for a leadership role such as partnership. This is understandable; it is difficult to ignore your gut instinct when evaluating other people. Recent advances in psychology, however, are shedding light on how traits evolve and even change. Over the past few decades more and more psychologists have challenged the assumption that we are born with a set of predetermined traits. For example, a branch of psychology called attribution theory has demonstrated that the 'mindsets' which determine our behaviour are much more learned (i.e. acquired) than had been originally assumed. It has been shown that people learn different reasons (or *attributions*) why certain events turned out as they did. Seligman and Maier (1967) have demonstrated how people 'learn to become helpless' when they assume, erroneously, that their circumstances are beyond their control. This is the basis of Seligman's theory of learned helplessness. While this theory and others like it (Dweck, 2000) were originally focused on resilience and well-being, the view that many of our key 'traits' are learned, as opposed to genetic, is also being applied to leadership (see below). As a result, most researchers no longer ask 'Can leadership be learned?' Rather, they are asking 'How is leadership learned?'

The skills approach

In contrast to the traits approach, the skills approach focuses on a leader's areas of competence as opposed to their personality. Katz's (1955) 'three-skill' model represents the classic approach to the skills-based theory of leadership and management. According to Katz, effective management and leadership depend on three essential areas of competence: technical, human and conceptual. Katz asserts that the relative importance of each varies between different management levels. For example, lower

(or supervisory) managers require mainly technical and human skill; middle managers require a significant component of all three, whereas upper management levels require higher levels of conceptual and human skill. In other words, the higher the leadership position, the greater the challenge of getting members of the group to work effectively together towards a common goal. Leaders therefore need increasing levels of 'human' and 'conceptual' competences to address this challenge as their level of leadership increases. A key premise of Katz's model is that since skills are 'learned' behaviours leadership is open to anyone motivated enough to develop the breadth of skills that enables them to get people to work together towards desirable future goals. This view is in contrast to the Great Man and earlier trait models, which assume leaders are a select group fortunate enough to be born with the right characteristics.

This model can be applied to both traditional veterinary practices and corporate groups. Assistant veterinary surgeons working in traditional independent practices often follow Katz's model of leadership development as they progress towards partnership. For example, they may become the 'core vet' at a branch surgery when they take on sole-charge responsibilities. This could be likened to a lower-level management position whereby they are in charge of the day-to-day technical and service operations, without having a say in higher management decisions such as purchasing decisions, pricing or profit objectives. Leading a branch is a very useful training ground for partnership as it helps a vet 'prove' their technical competences as well as their ability to deal with common 'people' issues. 'Common people issues' in veterinary practice often means getting on with the range of personalities and skill sets that are commonly found within the practice as well as an ability to resolve common client complaints.

Middle managers are common in many corporate veterinary chains in the form of territory managers who oversee a group of practices. Middle managers represent a crucial link between the staff working at the customer interface and the 'central' corporate managers. They therefore require at least some understanding of clinical systems in order to understand the impact of changing operational protocols. They also require enough people skills to communicate effectively with the vets, nurses, receptionists and administrators. In order for corporate strategies to be understood, adopted and implemented successfully, middle managers also need a higher level of business management knowledge (conceptual skills) than lower-level managers. For example, they need to be able to read and produce budgets as well as have an understanding of how their behaviour affects other commercial objectives.

Top-level managers within corporate practices, however, require a much deeper understanding of the conceptual models, systems and strategies which are central to commercial enterprises, irrespective of the particular industry in which they happen to be working. Technical competences are therefore less important at this level because clinical matters will be managed by the veterinary surgeons in the practices. Instead, they need to be able to blend their conceptual knowledge with well-developed people skills in order to communicate, persuade and negotiate effectively with various stakeholders, especially financiers, key suppliers and the middle managers, with whom they work. Traditionally, an MBA (Masters in Business Administration) has been seen as the higher-level management qualification whereby aspiring upper-level managers learn these skills. It is, of course, possible to act as a senior executive in any organization without any formal business qualifications, as many self-made entrepreneurs have demonstrated.

While the skills model may help us understand which of the basic minimal competencies people in veterinary businesses need in order to be effective as managers within their organizations, it does not always follow that having these skills automatically results in effective team work in pursuit of a common goal. This is because the skills model does not address the impact of values and ethics within the organization. Indeed, it

is entirely possible for two people with exactly the same skills and competencies to have entirely different opinions about a particular situation and the action that needs to be taken. For example, managers whose career progression depends on delivering good financial results may not always see eye to eye with veterinary clinical staff whose priority is to resolve clinical issues with less regard for profitability.

The behavioural or styles approach to leadership and management

The main thrust of the 'styles' approach is that leaders and managers prefer to behave in some ways rather than others. This is in contrast to the traits approach (which leaders possess) and the skills approach (which they have learnt).

The most well-known 'styles' model of leadership is Blake and Mouton's managerial grid (subsequently referred to as the Leadership Grid; Blake and Mouton, 1964, 1978, 1985). This model has been used extensively in many different organizational settings for training and development. To the author's knowledge, however, it has not been directly applied to the veterinary profession as a means of helping veterinary leaders address the leadership challenge (teamwork and purpose) within veterinary practice.

Blake and Mouton's Leadership Grid juxtaposes a leader's concern for production against their concern for people, in a two-by-two matrix as shown in Figure 4.1. The first plot point refers to a leader's

Figure 4.1 • A summary of leadership styles originally described in the Blake and Mouton Managerial Grid (adapted from Blake and Mouton, 1964)

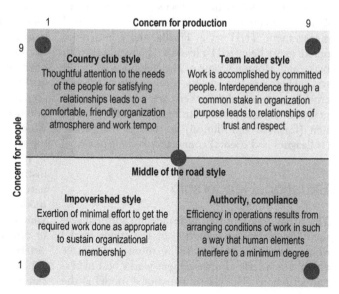

	Concern for production	
1		9

Country club style
Thoughtful attention to the needs of the people for satisfying relationships leads to a comfortable, friendly organization atmosphere and work tempo

Team leader style
Work is accomplished by committed people. Interdependence through a common stake in organization purpose leads to relationships of trust and respect

Middle of the road style

Impoverished style
Exertion of minimal effort to get the required work done as appropriate to sustain organizational membership

Authority, compliance
Efficiency in operations results from arranging conditions of work in such a way that human elements interfere to a minimum degree

Concern for people

orientation towards production (i.e. outcome tasks), and the second plot point refers to their orientation towards people or employees. While any combination of plots is possible, Blake and Mouton identify five 'classic' leadership styles: authority-compliance (9,1), country-club management (1,9), impoverished management (1,1), middle-of-the-road management (5,5) and team leader (9,9).

Within the veterinary profession, 'concern for production' can be likened to a preference for certain performance indicators such as clinical or financial outcomes. 'Concern for people', however, reflects the degree to which the practice leader cares about his or her team's morale, client engagement and satisfaction. In the author's experience, it is possible to categorize leaders of practices within the UK into each of the five stereotypical styles described in this model. Some bosses are much more authoritarian and imposing than others with respect to achieving certain targets (often financial) in ways that constrain autonomy with respect to clinical decision-making. This could be likened to the 'authority-compliance' (9,1) style. Veterinary corporate organizations are sometimes 'accused' of having this style of leadership. In the author's experience, however, corporate groups are no more likely to exhibit this style of leadership than independently owned practices, some of which can also be quite authoritarian. The 'country-club management' (1,9) style is less common although it does exist. Some veterinary practices in the UK are run with much more concern for team morale than the practice's financial or even technical level of performance. In contrast, some practices seem to lack any particular focus – performance or social – and could be described as the 'impoverished management' (1,1) style. Finally, more and more practices are being led by leaders who would fit with Blake and Mouton's view of the 'team leader' (9,9) style. These practice leaders, some of whom are veterinary partners while others are non-veterinarian practice managers, have a strong concern for production (financial and clinical) as well as the people (colleagues and clients) connected to their practice.

Situational leadership

The situational approach to leadership and management represents an evolution of the styles model described above. It aims to be more prescriptive about which style of management works best in certain situations. The classic situational model is the Hersey–Blanchard model, which advocates that a leader's style should depend on the level of maturity of the members within the group. This theory is based on the premise that leadership is composed of both directive and supportive dimensions. Directive behaviour is the extent to which a leader explicitly commands group members to carry out certain duties in pursuit of a specific goal. Supportive behaviour is the extent to which a leader engages in two-way communication with the aim of providing socio-emotional 'support' in order to get the members of the group to work effectively together. Maturity is conceptualized as the willingness and the ability of the group members to take responsibility for selecting specific goals as well as the means of accomplishing them. Blanchard asserts that by assessing the maturity level of the followers in relation to a specific task, a leader or manager can choose to adopt one of four styles: supporting, coaching, delegating or directing. As the level of followers' maturity increases, the manager reduces his or her directive behaviour and increases his or her supportive behaviour. As the followers' level of maturity develops further, the leader should decrease both directive and supportive behaviour.

A veterinary career could be described as a series of transitions ranging from pre-graduation through to retirement, and each stage has its own challenges and rewards. The situational leadership model provides an easily understood, easily applied set of 'prescriptive' behaviours as to how veterinary managers and leaders should adapt their behaviours in relation to the career stage of their staff. The model applies equally well to clinical staff as it does to lower or middle managerial staff members. In a clinical capacity, for example, the directing style is often adopted with unqualified assistants, such as student veterinary nurses or even veterinary undergraduates. Aspects of the coaching style would be applicable to a newly qualified veterinary surgeon in their first year, progressing to a supporting style as confidence and competence increase, resulting in higher independence, which in turn results in the transition to the delegating style.

It is likely that many veterinary managers do this instinctively as they work alongside the newer graduates they manage or employ. The challenge with this model, however, is to know which situations and which team members require more or less supportive or directive input. For example, the wide range of veterinary tasks as well as the degree to which different personalities invite or resist direction and support can make this decision difficult.

Table 4.2 A summary of some of the key characteristics of transformational leaders originally described by Bass in 1985

Idealized influence

Transformational leaders are guided by a sense of purpose and values, and consider the moral and ethical consequences of their decisions. As well as championing exciting new possibilities, they talk about the importance of trusting each other and going beyond their self-interests for the good of the group. They act in ways that build respect as well as exhibiting a sense of power and competence, which reassures others that obstacles can be overcome

Inspirational motivation

Transformational leaders talk optimistically about the future and about what needs to be accomplished. They articulate a compelling vision and an exciting image of what is essential to consider, as well as expressing confidence that goals will be achieved. Their strong sense of values enables them to take a stand on controversial issues

Intellectual stimulation

This is the ability to identify and examine critical assumptions as well as questioning whether they are appropriate. Transformational leaders will readily seek different perspectives when solving problems, as well as getting others to look at problems from many different angles in order to find new ways of looking at how to deal with traditional problems. They spend time teaching and coaching, and treat others as individuals rather than just as members of a group by considering their different needs, abilities and aspirations

Individualized consideration

This is the ability to help others develop their strengths, listen attentively to their concerns and find ways to promote their development

Source: adapted from Bass (1985).

Transactional and transformational leadership

Transactional versus transformational views of management and leadership have been proposed as another way of explaining the difference between leadership and management (Bass, 1985; Burns, 1978). The transactional approach refers to the exchange that occurs between managers and their group in return for rewards and promotions. The transformational approach, however, is a process whereby the leader aims to connect with members of the group in a way that transforms their outlook and uplifts them. This model of leadership describes how leaders use emotions, values, ethics, standards and long-term goals to get the members of their group to work effectively together in pursuit of a common goal. Burns asserts that leaders need to exhibit a degree of each of the following four key characteristics if they wish to act as transformational leaders (Bass, 1985; Burns, 1978), as summarized in Table 4.2.

A key strength of this model is its future orientation and sense of purpose. This model also portrays the image of an 'idealized' role model who gets his or her followers to work effectively together in pursuit of engaging goals. With respect to the veterinary profession, the transformational model of leadership resonates well with the traditional image of the wise, experienced and even benevolent veterinary partner who projects a clear sense of morals, values and ethical conduct and inspires others to do likewise. It could also be used to describe any enthusiastic 'personality' working within veterinary practice who personifies a range of good outcomes such as good patient and client care, commercial contribution and team harmony. It is these types of 'inspiring' characters, many of whom perform leadership roles within their practice, who are generally celebrated in the annual Petplan Veterinary Awards. While this concept of leadership is intuitively very appealing, it could be challenged on the basis that the leader's ability to display the four key characteristics of transformational leadership listed above is contingent on possessing and displaying certain personality 'traits'. It could also be argued that it is entirely possible to unite a team of people in pursuit of a common goal without having all or even any of these characteristics. Furthermore, the model, as Burns and Bass describe it, is more descriptive than prescriptive in orientation and lacks specifics about how aspiring leaders develop and transfer their own sense of enthusiasm, purpose, standards and ethics on to those they wish to 'transform'.

The cultural approach

Culture is defined as 'a pattern of shared basic assumptions that the group learned as it solved its problems of external adaptation and internal integration that has worked well enough to be considered valid and therefore, to be taught to new members as the correct way to perceive, think, and feel in relation to those problems' (Schein, 2004). In other words, we all live within groups (nations, workplaces, families, clubs, etc.) which teach us to believe that there are right and wrong ways of dealing with problems and achieving good outcomes. We are not born with opinions about what is good or bad, right or wrong; rather, we acquire them as we go through life when we learn what goals are worth striving for and why, as well as how we should go about achieving them. We learn our beliefs from the people we spend time with and through the experiences we share. It is important to realize, however, that 'right and wrong' and 'good and bad' are subjective terms. What one person or one group believes to be a 'good' outcome may not be considered 'good' by another. Similarly, what one group believes is the 'right' way to do something, may be considered 'wrong' by another. Culture (i.e. what groups of people believe is 'right or wrong', 'good or bad') therefore acts as a set of social 'forces' which help members of that group know where they stand in relation to what behaviours and standards are acceptable, rejected or encouraged. Culture gives people a template of how to interpret the world as well as a sense of how to respond when certain things happen. This template makes the 'world' meaningful and predictable by helping us contain the anxiety that comes from chaos and uncertainty. In other words, people feel more secure, reassured and in control of social situations when they have a strong sense about what others see as the 'right and wrong ways of going about achieving good or bad outcomes'. They may not always agree with their group's agenda or methods, but at least they know where they stand in relation to them.

The process of creating and managing a group's culture has been described as the essence of leadership (Schein, 2004). In other words, Schein believes that it is impossible to consider leadership without considering culture, since a group's beliefs about 'right and wrong, good and bad' (i.e. its culture) originate from the founder's own sense of 'right and wrong, good and bad'. If the group is successful the leader's opinions will be adopted, shared and taken for granted by its members 'as the right way to do things'. Group members who do not agree with the leader's goals and values may enter into a 'power struggle' with them or alternatively leave the organization. While managers may monitor and measure how well an organization is achieving its stated objectives, leaders decide what those objectives are (i.e. what defines a good outcome) and often how they should be achieved (i.e. what is the right way to go about doing things). Schein (2004) asserts that it is essential for leaders to achieve a critical level of consensus about right and wrong, good and bad, if they wish to unite their team in pursuit of a common goal. It is therefore essential that leaders understand the nature of the invisible psychological forces at play

within their group if they want to harness them to achieve their objectives.

The cultural model is particularly applicable to understanding the dynamics within veterinary practice. Veterinary organizations often have a range of purposes including resolution and prevention of disease and suffering, profit generation and acting as vehicles for personal and professional fulfilment. By interpreting leadership in terms of beliefs about 'good and bad, right and wrong', we can begin to understand why different practices advocate different operational protocols and behaviours, as well as why such protocols may or may not be adopted.

The cultural model of leadership can also help explain why leaders face a greater challenge when there is a wider cultural diversity between members within an organization. For example, this model helps us understand the tension that can exist between veterinary surgeons and non-veterinary managers. Clinicians are motivated to understand and resolve the conundrum of animal disease because of the intellectual and physical challenge required. They also take a professional oath, which obligates them to act as the guardians against animal suffering and distress. In contrast, managers in veterinary organizations are ultimately employed to represent their shareholders' interests. While many non-veterinary managers may, of course, share a personal empathy for animal welfare, they also have a legal obligation to maximize profit on behalf of the shareholders they represent. This does not necessarily mean that these different objectives and obligations are irreconcilable. It does, however, highlight the challenge that leaders of these organizations face if they are to create and manage a culture which adapts and succeeds in a commercial sense, while at the same time maintaining consensus with regard to how everyone in the organization defines 'good outcomes' and how to achieve them.

The difference between the cultural model and the transformational model of leadership is that the cultural model recognizes the need for a 'consensual' relationship between leaders and followers that is grounded in common values, beliefs and expectations about goals and behaviour. Schein's (2004) cultural model of leadership helps leaders understand the impact of their own assumptions, beliefs and behaviours on the group, and vice versa. A crucial feature of this model is that in order for a leader to address the two main challenges of leadership, which have been the main theme of this chapter (teamwork and purpose), they must recognize and manage the connection between the group's subconscious beliefs and their observable behaviour. In other words, leaders need to be aware of how a group's collective beliefs evolve through shared experiences and subsequently act as a psychological 'blueprint' that guides and constrains the group's motives and behaviours.

Conclusions

The literature on leadership is vast. This in part reflects a lack of consensus about what leadership actually is and what specific issues it aims to address. Ultimately, there is a lack of specific evidence-based studies examining how each of the leadership models discussed here relates to leadership within the veterinary profession. The aim of this chapter, therefore, was to give the reader an insight into the variety of leadership models that have been used within other business and political arenas.

There is a consensus that management and leadership are diverse concepts and that they do not mean the same thing to everyone. While leadership is sometimes referred to as if it is simply 'advanced management', it is perhaps more useful to think of 'leaders' and 'managers' as two distinct modes of operating, with entirely different levels of focus and scope.

Leadership can be conceptualized and investigated at various different levels. These range from the more externally observable or 'tangible' dimensions of leadership, as described in the traits, skills and styles approaches, to the more intangible or psychological

levels as described in the transformational and cultural models.

The more externally observable models of leadership have traditionally leant towards the assumption that leaders are born, not made. In contrast, the more psychological models of leadership argue that leadership is something that can be learnt by understanding the mental 'systems' that connect our collective assumptions, values, beliefs and behaviours.

Summary

This chapter has distinguished between the concepts of management and leadership, and has explored the various leadership styles discussed in the literature. A number of leadership theories and models were presented and compared. The importance of leadership in the veterinary context was emphasized, with the conclusion that some of the models of leadership discussed can be learnt.

Review questions

1. What is the difference between management and leadership?
2. What is the purpose of leadership?
3. What do leaders do that makes them effective?
4. How do leaders think? What do they think about?
5. Which leadership models make most sense to you?

References

Bass, B.M., 1985. Leadership and Performance: Beyond Expectation. Free Press, New York.

Bass, B.M., 1990. Bass and Stogdill's Handbook of Leadership: A Survey of Theory and Research. Free Press, New York.

Bennis, W.G., Naus, B., 1985. Leaders: The Strategies for Taking Charge. Harper & Row, New York.

Blake, R.R., Mouton, J.S., 1964. The Managerial Grid: The Key to Leadership Excellence. Gulf, Houston, TX.

Blake, R.R., Mouton, J.S., 1978. The New Managerial Grid. Gulf, Houston, TX.

Blake, R.R., Mouton, J.S., 1985. The Managerial Grid III. Gulf, Houston, TX.

Burns, J.M., 1978. Leadership. Harper & Row, New York.

Costa, P.T., McCrae, R.R., 1994. 'Set like plaster?' Evidence for the stability of adult personality. In: Heatheton, T., Weinberger, J. (Eds.), Can Personality Change? American Psychological Association, Washington, DC, pp. 21–40.

Dweck, C.S., 2000. Self Theories: Their Role in Motivation, Personality and Development. Psychology Press, New York.

Eysenck, H.J., 1982. Personality, Genetics and Behaviour. Praeger, New York.

Goldberg, L.R., 1990. An alternative 'description' of personality: the big-five factor structure. J.

Pers. Soc. Psychol. 59, 1216–1299.

Jago, A.G., 1982. Leadership: perspectives in theory and research. Management Science 28 (3), 315–336.

Kassin, S., 2003. Psychology. Prentice Hall, Upper Saddle River, NJ.

Katz, R.L., 1955. Skills of an effective administrator. Harv. Bus. Rev. 33 (1), 33–42.

Kirkpatrick, S.A., Locke, E.A., 1991. Leadership: do traits matter? The Executive 5, 48–60.

Kotter, J.P., 1990. A Force of Change: How Leadership Differs from Management. Free Press, New York.

Little, G., 2011. Taking the lead: heading a team successfully. In Pract. 33, 138–140.

Loehlin, J.C., 1992. Genes and Environment and Personality Development. Sage, Newbury Park, CA.

Lord, R.G., DeVader, C.L., Alliger, G.M., 1986. A meta-analysis of the relation between personality traits and leadership perceptions: an application of validity generalization procedures. J. Appl. Psychol. 71, 402–410.

McCrae, R.R., John, O.P., 1992. An introduction to the five-factor and its applications. J. Pers. 60, 175–215.

Northouse, P.G., 2010. Leadership: Theory and Practice, fifth ed. Sage, Thousand Oaks, CA.

Rost, J.C., 1991. Leadership for the Twenty First Century. Praeger, New York.

Schein, E.H., 2004. Organizational Culture and Leadership. Jossey-Bass, San Francisco, CA.

Seligman, M.E., Maier, S.F., 1967. Failure to escape electric shock. J. Exp. Psychol. 74, 1–9.

Sheridan, J.P., McCafferty, O.E., 1993. The Business of Veterinary Practice. Pergamon Press, Oxford.

Stogdill, R.M., 1948. Personal factors associated with leadership: a survey of the literature. J. Psychol. 25, 35–71.

Stogdill, R.M., 1974. Handbook of Leadership: A Survey of Theory and Research. Free Press, New York.

Zaccaro, S.J., Kemp, C., Bader, P., 2004. Leader traits and attributes. In: Antonakis, J., Cianciola, A.T., Sternberg, R.J. (Eds.), The Nature of Leadership. Sage, Thousand Oaks, CA, pp. 101–124.

Veterinary business management: an ethical approach to managing people and practices

5

Lorna Treanor   Martin Whiting

CHAPTER OVERVIEW

This chapter introduces students to the ethical management of people and practices, highlighting the knowledge and skills that employers and the Royal College of Veterinary Surgeons (RCVS) expect from new graduates, and provides an insight into what they might expect as an employee. Human resource management (HRM) practice within veterinary businesses is outlined with special consideration given to the motivation, training and development of all practice staff, including veterinary nurses. Key theories and concepts of ethics, professionalism and management are introduced to students, with both good and poor practice examples used to illustrate possible practical issues that may arise in the workplace.

LEARNING OUTCOMES

After reading this chapter, students will be able to:
- Demonstrate an understanding of the wider veterinary business context.
- Define the key functions of management and evaluate the appropriateness of different management styles in different situations and contexts.
- Identify key motivation theories and understand their relationship to HRM.
- Appreciate the relevant RCVS Day One Competence expectations for graduate veterinarians in the workplace in relation to ethics, professionalism and business acumen.
- Identify and critically appraise the ethical and professional expectations of a veterinary graduate working in practice.

Introduction

The veterinary profession has undergone dramatic changes over the past forty years. There is now a greater focus on animal welfare; large-animal work has declined while small or companion animal practice has increased (Lowe, 2009). There has also been a gender shift amongst veterinarians in practice, and different business models now operate within the veterinary business landscape (Henry and Treanor, 2012; RCVS, 2010). Traditionally, the profession was comprised of small, privately owned, partnership practices. In the UK, these are increasingly being taken over or replaced by corporate chains or groups of larger practices (Henry et al., 2011). This trend, coupled with the introduction of practices owned or managed by non-veterinarians, has created concerns that the 'managerialization' of the profession could result in practice 'unbecoming of the profession', should profit maximization concerns overtake healthcare decisions based on the patient's (animal's) best interests. There are additional concerns that sales and marketing strategies employed within some practices may diminish professional status by reducing veterinarians to sales staff, striving to achieve monthly targets.

In a challenging economic climate and an increasingly competitive veterinary business landscape, financial sustainability is difficult. As employers, practice owners are seeking graduates with business acumen – one of the 'Day One Competence' requirements of the RCVS. However, it has been claimed that UK veterinary graduates are insufficiently prepared for working in practice, unaware of the

© 2014, Elsevier Ltd.

business environment and, despite the fact that most will probably work within or lead a small veterinary business at some stage in their careers, ill prepared for management or leadership roles (Lowe, 2009). As a new employee, management responsibilities are unlikely; however, after a relatively short period of time, many veterinary graduates may find themselves adopting informal management roles as they become more experienced veterinary assistants, especially within smaller practices. These roles could range from the smaller-scale management of the veterinary team in animal care cases, through to the management of independent revenue streams from particular service offerings or areas of veterinary work within the overall practice. Unfortunately, many veterinarians in the workplace may not appreciate the benefits of undertaking management training, even when they become business owners and have responsibility for employees. The RCVS (2010) survey data highlight that time spent on practice management and administration is reported to have steadily increased between 2001 and 2010, with this trend forecast to continue. Additionally, a negative experience in a graduate's first post can dramatically shape their veterinary career, often triggering an early exit from the profession (Heath, 2007; RCVS, 2007). These studies have also highlighted the limited adoption of human resource (HR) practices, such as appraisals, that could make a positive contribution to the training, development and support of new graduates (RCVS, 2007, 2010).

This chapter introduces students to concepts relevant to the management of people and veterinary practices within a framework of ethics consistent with the profession; it is thus divided into two sections. The first section introduces business ethics before outlining core management theories. In the context of the ethical management of people, it focuses on human resource management, outlining HR management practices and techniques that new veterinarians may encounter in the workplace. Motivation theories are discussed to facilitate identification of personal motivational factors that can aid effective management of personal and career development, as well as providing an insight into appropriate management styles and approaches available to students when managing others in the veterinary team.

Given that ethical business management relies upon compliant behaviour of employees, the final section in the chapter introduces the expectations from graduate veterinarians from both the UK's veterinary regulatory body (RCVS) and prospective employers. Throughout the section the text highlights, using examples, the potential ethical and business tensions and challenges faced by veterinary practice owners and veterinarians working in practice.

Business ethics

Business ethics is a branch of applied ethics that 'addresses the moral features of commercial activity' (Marcoux, 2008). 'In particular, it involves examining appropriate constraints on the pursuit of self-interest, or (for firms) profits, when the actions of individuals or firms affect others' (MacDonald, 2012).

Recently, business ethics has explored financial accounting standards and practices, e.g. the Enron scandal or unscrupulous investment banking. Other concerns have also been raised, such as environmental issues due to corporations abusing the world's physical resources and causing environmental and ecological damage (Esso); abuse of human rights, e.g. Shell in Nigeria; and animal welfare, e.g. KFC and McDonalds (McDonalds v Steel & Morris, 1997; Rose, 2007). Unethical HRM practice has also been highlighted, e.g. the use of child labour by the fashion industry or employers reneging on pension agreements.

Business ethics in professional subjects, especially healthcare, are particularly problematic. One defining trait of a professional subject is the possession and application of the subject's unique body of knowledge; this distinguishes it from other business ethics as clients are unable to understand fully the role of the professional practitioner. Clients must invest a high level of trust in the professional to deliver fair, honest and appropriate information to them, not limiting their choices or freedom and acting altruistically for the best interests of the individuals involved. When the choices to be made relate to healthcare they are more significant and intense, especially if the decisions involve life-shortening or serious compromises on welfare. A broader view of business morality is required in considering the role of corporate responsibility in society, as evidenced by the RCVS's new Code of Professional Conduct for Veterinary Surgeons (RCVS, 2012a). The professional identity of veterinarians is so important that if one is to be employed by an organization then the RCVS recommends that the organization not only allows veterinarians to adhere to their professional conduct, but also makes sure that they are appointed to director status, ensuring that the professional conduct of the business aligns with RCVS expectations (RCVS, 2012b, Section 17.5).

An understanding of ethical approaches and considerations when managing people and practices is important for new veterinarians both as employees and practitioners. As a new employee, transitioning from student to professional, working within a complex business environment, new graduates can benefit from an understanding of the expectations their employers and the profession's regulators have of them.

Part I: Management theory

Management, like veterinary medicine, is considered to be part *art* and part *science*; while some individuals will have natural aptitudes, there are skills, knowledge and behaviours that can be taught and learned by all. Henri Fayol (1949) considered management to be a primarily intellectual activity that, regardless of the type of business, involved four core functions: planning, leading, organizing and controlling. At a macro level within a practice, the owner(s) will undertake these tasks to manage the business in its wider business environment. At the micro level, veterinarians will perform these tasks when managing care in each individual animal patient case.

Planning refers to anticipating future changes, identifying appropriate courses of action and then selecting the most appropriate course. The practice owner must anticipate changes within the wider business environment that could impact upon their business, including: customer expectations, competitors, the economic climate, government legislation or developments in technology. Having appraised the business environment, owner-managers must then set business objectives – statements of what needs done and by when – and devise operational plans to realize those objectives, regularly monitoring progress. In a veterinary practice, owners must stay abreast of the availability of cheaper generic drugs, new regulations from the RCVS, competitors opening branches close to their premises, competitor pricing and promotions, changes to insurance company coverage or claim procedures.

Leading involves communicating and fostering a shared vision for the business, supervising and motivating employees to work towards achieving that vision through achieving the business objectives. Fayol considered it imperative that managers understand employees in order to motivate them. He also advocated managers leading by example and treating employees appropriately and consistently, in line with the policies and structures of the business. Extensive research into motivation and leadership has informed good management practice from job design to communication, through to remuneration and staff training and development. These are elements of management that fall under the remit of an HRM function within larger organizations; in a small business environment, it is often an additional task undertaken by a general manager, such as a veterinarian.

Organizing involves ensuring the necessary logistical elements are in place to implement plans and deliver objectives. This would include ordering sufficient medicines and consumables to ensure treatment is possible through to recruiting, evaluating and training staff, setting working hours and devising work rotas, and ensuring procedures, processes and structures are in place to enable people to work effectively, safely and lawfully. From the perspective of good staff management, job design and preparing job descriptions, allocating staff responsibilities and roles all come under the umbrella of organizing. Research into job design has identified that over-specialization, reducing a job to one very small task, can have negative consequences on employee morale and motivation; people like to have autonomy and variety in their work. Just as new graduate veterinarians would quickly become demotivated if they were to undertake only cat spays every day, veterinary nurses too will want freedom to utilize their skill sets in order to remain motivated.

Controlling involves keeping plans and progress under review in order to identify and react to unexpected contingencies or to identify poor performance and take corrective action. Quality standards would also be monitored and, where necessary, corrective measures taken.

While this depicts management as a linear, logical and timely activity as opposed to a process that is undertaken with limited information and short timescales, it does outline the main aspects of management, and the importance of people, in having a successful business. While these may be the basic functions that managers must perform in their role, the manner in which these are conducted will produce different outcomes.

Management styles

People have a natural tendency to act and make decisions in a particular way; this is their natural management style. However, the management style adopted by a manager will impact upon the motivation and productivity of employees. Sometimes, when managing particular individuals or circumstances, managers may have to adopt a style with which they are less comfortable in order to achieve the best results. The main management styles are outlined in Box 5.1.

Human resource management

HRM can be considered as a 'business function that is concerned with managing relations between groups of people in their capacities as employees, employers and managers' (Rose, 2007). HRM involves attracting, selecting and retaining (through appraisal, training and development, remuneration and team building) the right people for each post. It also

involves ensuring compliance with employment legislation, dealing with whistle-blowing incidents and, where applicable, liaising and negotiating with unions. Today, HR is considered to have four objectives: (1) aligning HR and business strategy (strategic partner); (2) re-engineering organization processes (administration expert); (3) listening and responding to employees (employee champion); and (4) managing transformation and change (change agent) (Ulrich, 1996). While it may seem like a mixture of common sense and professional and legislative demands, HR practice today is informed by a long history of research into human motivation and organizational behaviour, in addition to attitudinal changes in society over time.

Management theory and motivation

Frederick Taylor (1911) sought to improve labour efficiency in a manufacturing plant; his work began what became known as the 'school of scientific management'. This approach advocated an autocratic

---

Box 5.1

Management/leadership styles

- Autocratic/authoritarian

   This can be a highly effective management style when employed in appropriate circumstances. An authoritarian style is characterized by a senior manager who takes all decisions and issues orders to staff. If this style is adopted in deciding all issues from the annual staff party to business development, it will usually result in a demotivated workforce. However, in emergency and critical care situations within veterinary surgery when there is an admission requiring surgery urgently, time is critical and clear instructions may be required to ensure everyone knows the treatment method being adopted and what they are expected to do, this would be a highly effective and appropriate management style in these circumstances.

- Democratic/participative

   In allowing team members to input into the decision-making process, the manager can benefit from the skills, perspectives and creativity of other team members and will often generate better ideas and plans as a result. While the manager will ultimately shape the decision-making process, this approach reinforces both 'team spirit' and an understanding of the shared business objectives that everyone should be working towards. Employees tend to be more motivated when their feedback is sought and this can also create greater 'buy-in' for the final decisions and

plans that are made. This style could be used by the same manager when deciding on appropriate marketing and advertising for the practice, for example.

- Laissez-faire

   A laissez-faire or hands-off management approach is characterized by team members being given autonomy and authority to a much greater extent. This approach allows greater potential for underperformance and staff could become demotivated if they mistook the hands-off approach as a lack of interest on behalf of the manager. If the manager wants to successfully employ this approach they should also employ an 'open door' policy so that employees know that support is readily available. Additionally, a coaching or mentoring approach would mean that individuals feel fully supported to develop and perform. This management style might be appropriate should the registered veterinary nurse be given responsibility and autonomy for certain clinics, such as obesity, behaviour or client follow-up. However, regular reporting or review of the outcomes should be undertaken to assess effectiveness of these clinics as a business model and identify other possible avenues to build customer loyalty and generate income. Delegation does not equate to dereliction of responsibility or authority from the management team.

management style (whereby managers make decisions and simply give orders to those below them). This style was later (1960) identified by McGregor as a theory X[1] style, i.e. managers regarded workers as lazy, requiring close supervision and motivated by pay. In scientific management, work was broken down into small chunks with people trained to perform a particular task. Jobs were repetitive in nature and 'time and motion' studies established normative work rates. Henry Ford used these concepts when establishing the first production line.

The work of Elton Mayo (the Hawthorne studies) in the 1920s showed that factors other than money determined worker productivity. The fact that management was showing an interest in employees' working conditions was found to motivate employees to achieve higher performance. Mayo also found that increased management–employee communication, in particular the opportunity for employees to give feedback, and having employees work in groups or teams, also significantly improved employee motivation and positively impacted upon expected productivity rates. This became the basis for the 'human relations school' of management.

Research into work motivation and the field of organizational behaviour gained momentum. In psychology, motivation is an explanatory concept used to describe why individuals behave in certain ways. Motivation itself is intrinsic to an individual and cannot be bestowed upon employees by managers; motivation is, however, affected by extrinsic rewards (tangible benefits such as pay, pensions, fringe benefits), intrinsic rewards (psychological rewards from doing the work itself, being part of an organization, profession or team, a sense of challenge or achievement) and social rewards (obtained by being with other people, sharing a sense of purpose, confirmation of identity and image of self) (Rollinson et al., 2002). This neo-human relations school of management focused on the psychological needs of employees and was heavily influenced by Abraham Maslow (1943, 1954) and Frederick Herzberg et al. (1959).

Maslow identified five levels of needs that people seek to satisfy. These needs are organized into a hierarchy to reflect that, as one type of need is largely satisfied, the next higher level of need begins to act as a

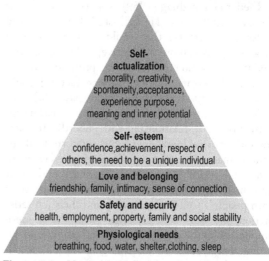

Figure 5.1 • Maslow's hierarchy of needs.
Based on data from Maslow, A. H. (1954). Motivation and personality. New York: Harper.

motivator (Figure 5.1). As physical and safety needs are met in a modern workplace, an employee may want to establish social networks to achieve a sense of belonging. If employees feel that their work is appreciated and valued by their employer, perhaps through promotion, pay and praise, they may be more motivated by an intrinsic drive for self-actualization, i.e. personal growth and fulfilment. Movement through the hierarchy is not one directional; people can move up and down the hierarchy as changes occur in their home or working lives.

The key implication of this theory for managers is that different people are motivated by a variety of different things, and what motivates an individual may change over time. Therefore, offering a range of benefits and incentives can motivate staff. For example, some large organizations operate a 'cafeteria-style' benefit plan allowing employees to choose the benefits they value most, e.g. pay, time off, a health plan or gym membership. Veterinarians would typically operate at the top end of Maslow's hierarchy. A practice manager should aim to support and motivate staff to level 5: self-actualization. HR practices such as appraisals and staff training and development e.g. continuing professional development (CPD) training, could play a major role in the continuing motivation of veterinarians as they may seek to improve their clinical and non-clinical skills, to have greater variety in their workload or wish to specialize and develop an expertise in a particular area.

---

[1] McGregor's theory X and Y of management reflects two opposing attitudes that managers hold about employees. Theory X is outlined above; theory Y is where managers consider workers to be self-motivated, ambitious, capable of self-control and motivated by the satisfaction of doing a good job.

Frederick Herzberg (1959) proposed a two-factor theory of motivation. He suggested that there were factors (motivators) that could be introduced to make employees more productive, including responsibility, recognition, achievement, promotion or the work itself. Other factors (hygiene factors) could demotivate employees: these include pay, work conditions, personal life, company policy, relationship with supervisor, relationship with subordinates, status and security. Herzberg (1959) supported a democratic management style where employees were consulted and able to provide feedback and input into the decision-making process. He was concerned with people's well-being at work and their job satisfaction; his work strongly aligns with the modern emphasis on ethical management and team building.

Herzberg promoted job enlargement, job enrichment and empowerment. Job enlargement is sometimes referred to as horizontal loading; a job is made more interesting for an employee by adding different tasks of a similar level of difficulty in order to provide some variety. Job enrichment is where additional tasks that are more challenging are added to a job; this can be considered as vertical enrichment. This may mean that one employee undertakes all aspects of completing a particular task, thus providing a greater sense of accomplishment. Care is required, however, to ensure that employees do not feel they are being given additional work with no reward.

Empowerment involves management delegating greater power and responsibility for work to employees, improving motivation by enabling them to become more autonomous and self-directed. In a veterinary context, giving the receptionist responsibility for client follow-up and vaccination reminders could add variety and responsibility to the job role while assisting the financial sustainability of the practice. Registered veterinary nurses are highly trained, committed team members who could be given responsibility for running dental or puppy clinics. Alternatively, a veterinarian could be given responsibility for establishing or developing a new service within the practice – for example, an arthritis clinic.

David McClelland's (1961) motivational needs theory was closely related to Herzberg's work. McClelland identified three types of motivational need (Box 5.2) which he proposed were found to varying degrees in all workers and managers. He suggested that the dominant need or needs within given individuals would influence their management style and behaviours, as well as affecting how they are

---

Box 5.2

McClelland's motivational needs

- Need for achievement

  Individuals with a high need for achievement are motivated by challenging but attainable goals and advancement within their job. They need a lot of feedback on their performance (Stahl, 1983) and seek a sense of accomplishment. They will be quite responsive to Herzberg's motivators. Achievers prefer to work with others they consider competent (Kirby, 2003); their preoccupation is succeeding in whatever they undertake and they find the prospects of failure highly depressing, and so engage in failure avoidance strategies (Rollinson and Broadfield, 2002). They often prefer to work alone so they can take full responsibility for what they do. They tend not to value money for itself but more as a symbol of success (Chusmir and Parker, 1992). As managers, these individuals can be very demanding of their staff; they will tend towards a theory X disposition and will prioritize task accomplishment.

- Need for authority and power

  Individuals with a high need for authority and power seek to be influential and have an impact. They will want to increase their personal status and prestige, seeking leadership roles. They are usually theory X in their management approach.

- Need for affiliation:

  People with a high need for affiliation are team players; they like friendly relationships with others and like to be popular with good workplace relations. Managers with a high need for affiliation tend to adopt a theory Y approach.

---

motivated and how they motivate others. The three motivational needs are illustrated in Box 5.2.

The work of Maslow, Herzberg and McClelland falls under what are termed *content* or *needs* theories of motivation. They are complementary in that they all assume that motivation is best understood by exploring the structure of innate or learned human needs. The 'process' theories of motivation also enable greater insight into employee motivation and behaviours. Process theories explicitly acknowledge that human needs provide the motivational impetus for action, but they focus on how these needs are translated into patterns of behaviour (Rollinson and Broadfield, 2002, p. 200). Process theories therefore aim to inform us as to *how* particular individuals come to be motivated.

The most widely known process theory of motivation is Vroom's (1964) expectancy theory. Essentially, this proposes that individuals are motivated to act if they

Motivational force = Expectancy × Instrumentality × Valence

Figure 5.2 • Vroom's expectancy theory

perceive they are likely to achieve an expected outcome that holds value for them. It is commonly expressed as an equation (Figure 5.2).

Expectancy is connected to the effort–performance relationship: an individual's belief that their effort/action will lead to the desired performance. The strength of expectancy will be directly affected by factors such as past experience, self-confidence and their perception of the difficulty of the performance goal. 'Instrumentality' relates to the performance–outcome relationship. It refers to the probability that, if you perform in a certain manner or take a particular course of action, you will attain the expected outcome. 'Valence' refers to the value attached to the particular outcome by the individual. Individuals will therefore decide how hard they will work, and to what standard, based on the value of the outcomes they expect to derive.

John Adams' 'equity theory' of motivation (Adams, 1965) contends that pay and conditions alone will not dictate motivation. Adams outlined the human tendency to evaluate how we are being treated in comparison with others, meaning our satisfaction is dependent upon our perception of fair treatment. If employees feel that they are being treated fairly or advantageously then they are more likely to be motivated and maintain or improve their performance. If they perceive that they are being treated unfavourably in comparison to others, they will be demotivated. As part of this process, individuals will assess the ratio of their personal inputs (for example, how hard they work, how qualified they are, how long they have been with the company) and outputs (their pay and benefit rewards and working conditions). They will then compare this to a chosen 'referent' or 'comparison other'. This could be themselves at an earlier stage in their career with the same or a different company, or it could be with a comparable colleague within or outside their current company. Individuals, for example, may be happy with their salary package until they learn that a colleague, whom they perceive to be as skilled and as hard-working as they are, earns a higher salary. Adams suggested that having undertaken a comparison and made an equity judgement, individuals would experience tensions and would be motivated to act to lessen the tension

experienced. The actions could be to modify inputs (for example, if feeling under-rewarded, an employee would reduce effort), modify outputs (for example, ask for a pay rise or promotion), modify perceptions of self or the referent other or change the person used as a referent in order to re-establish a perception of equity and reduce tension, or leave.

Process theories of motivation place different emphases on the importance of internal and external factors and the role that rewards play in the motivational process. However, they all stress the need to establish clear links between performance and reward and, if motivation is to be achieved and maintained, it is crucially important to consider the work environment. It is also important to consider the different personality types and motivational needs of individual staff members when allocating roles, responsibilities and building an effective team. Within the veterinary context, veterinarians are typically high achievers. Like registered veterinary nurses, they derive job satisfaction and a sense of achievement from their work; for many, this may be more important than salary and can help compensate for negative aspects of working in practice, such as on-call requirements.

HR tools and techniques

All HR practices have an ethical foundation. HR deals with the practical consequences of human behaviour.

Johnson (2003)

Modern human resource management advocates the use of a range of tools and techniques to boost employee motivation and performance. Those most relevant to new veterinary graduates will be performance appraisals, training and development and remuneration.

Appraisals

Performance appraisal is a commonly used HR tool that enables individual employees to reflect objectively on their performance, skills and knowledge in conjunction with their manager. The aim is to identify areas where employees are performing well and areas where they require support or additional training. This is a formal feedback mechanism that can also be used to set goals and objectives for the individual for the period of time until the next review. This can be an uncomfortable task for both parties, especially in a small business environment where the appraiser is untrained and/or inexperienced, and the appraisee may be defensive. As a result appraisals can often be delayed, rushed or not undertaken at all.

New graduates should, however nervously, want to gain feedback on their performance, to identify areas where they are performing well and to discover those areas where they feel less comfortable and would like to undertake additional training. This can help in identifying CPD courses and activities to boost confidence and skill levels in different clinical and non-clinical areas. The natural tendency for individuals is to focus on things they enjoy and so, without input from a manager, individuals may always tend to select CPD in their areas of personal interest and expertise when it would be more beneficial for their professional development to undertake training in an area of weakness. Similarly, the practice owner or manager may identify opportunities to develop the business and may encourage staff to undertake relevant CPD to be involved in this new work area. The identification of suitable training could reflect skills gaps and needs in the individual, or in the business. Unfortunately, research (Heath, 1996, 2007) indicates that many practices do not undertake regular staff appraisals; this can leave members of the veterinary team feeling demotivated as they do not receive feedback to enable them to improve, or to let them know that their contribution is valued. Appraisals, when undertaken in an appropriate and timely manner, can aid employee motivation at levels four and five in Maslow's hierarchy of needs and positively impact on the business.

Staff training and development

Staff training and development deficits should be identified as a result of the appraisal process in line with individual and business needs. RCVS requires that veterinarians initially undertake a year-long Professional Development Phase followed by a minimum of 35 annual CPD hours averaged over a floating three-year period (RCVS, 2012c). This is to ensure that veterinarians remain abreast of new developments in treatments, medicines and clinical techniques, and to ensure that they remain professionally competent in their practice of veterinary medicine. CPD can include reading journals, observing practice with more experienced staff or specialists, attending seminars or undertaking further accredited training courses.

Within veterinary practices, the development and enhancement of the roles of other team members would not only boost their individual morale but could also assist the financial sustainability of the practice and lessen the workload on overburdened veterinarians.

Remuneration

Remuneration refers to the total package of payment provided to an employee in return for their working according to agreed contract terms. It typically comprises the salary and, possibly, housing and transport but can include other benefits, e.g. pensions, commission, insurance (health, dental, income protection and/or life insurance, amongst others, may be offered), gym or other sports memberships.

Salary

In comparison with their human medicine counterparts, veterinarians' working hours are often not restricted by the European Working Time Directive, as many sign waivers as part of their contracts. Their remuneration, especially in consideration of hours worked, can seem relatively poor. There is great variety between different geographical areas, areas of veterinary practice and individual practices in terms of salary and benefits offered. An appreciation of motivation theory suggests that salary is more likely to be a 'hygiene' factor, demotivating staff if set at an inappropriately low level. New veterinary graduates will often accept that they will start on a lower salary but that this will increase as they gain post-qualification experience and perhaps undertake additional training. In a challenging economic landscape some employers may not be financially able to pay employees as much as they would like, given obtainable market rates for services in their locale and increasing competition from online pharmaceutical suppliers and larger chains able to benefit from group purchasing discounts.

Commission

Many businesses provide staff with a minimum salary that is then enhanced by commission based on performance, e.g. in a production line environment bonuses are earned when performance exceeds the daily or weekly targets; in a sales environment a percentage of sales may be earned as commission to encourage staff to try and sell goods and services to customers. It must be remembered that no individual tool or technique is innately good or bad of itself; it is in the detail of their implementation that the likelihood of positive or negative outcomes from these schemes can be influenced. However, this cannot be predetermined in isolation; the people and the individual decisions they may take based on their personal circumstances, motivations and value systems will also determine outcomes. For example, three salespeople on the same acceptable monthly flat-rate salary may react differently. One may be less motivated to sell as their basic needs are met; one is just as motivated to sell as they would be if sales commission accounted for a larger proportion of salary because he or she has a high need for achievement, and the third, even though basic needs are met, may still be tempted to engage in unscrupulous sales practices to secure an increased income.

While in many businesses offering incentives to motivate employees is commonplace, there are concerns that in a healthcare environment this could place undue pressure on the professional judgement of veterinarians and nurses. The concern relates to individuals being so incentivized by monetary rewards attached to performing particular tests or selling particular products that they behave in a way considered to be unprofessional. This is a particular concern should such financial bonuses become a substantial component of the remuneration package. If incentives were so attractive that it caused veterinarians to reconsider treatment options or promote sales of unnecessary consumables to obtain their bonus, this could compromise the primacy of the animal's best interests. The outcomes will be determined by the ethics of the individual. One suggestion (Cousquer, 2011) is for employers to use an incentivization scheme that would prevent coercion and restriction of informed choice. Such a scheme would involve the same monetary reward for the sale of goods or services, but the money would only be available to spend on professional development, meaning that animals would ultimately benefit from highly trained veterinarians' care.

Part II: The graduate veterinarian as an ethical, professional employee

An ethical business relies on ethically minded employees. There will be many expectations of a graduate veterinarian as a professional employee – some of those from the regulatory body (RCVS) and some from employers. While there will be significant overlap, there may also be areas of tension.

RCVS Day One Competences

As part of veterinary degree programmes in the UK, all undergraduates undertake professional studies, the minimum content of which is determined by the governing body's statutory duty to determine the 'standard of proficiency' and 'knowledge and skill' required to practise veterinary medicine in the UK. The knowledge and skill sets required are laid out as a list of Day One Competences (RCVS, 2006), which further extend after a year's professional development phase, to Year One Competences.

The Day One Competences from the RCVS outline the expected skill set from a new graduate entering the profession; these partly reflect employer expectations. These include generic skills, but also those that can be specifically translated into ethical business management (RCVS, 2006) (Box 5.3). All of these competences must be met and undertaken while conforming to the five core principles of practice as outlined in the Code of Professional Conduct for Veterinary Surgeons (RCVS, 2012a).

Ethical responsibilities (A1.4)

Day One Competences A1.4 and A1.5 relate to the image of a morally responsible professional. To understand the first, one must consider the ethical implications of how an individual undertakes the role of a veterinarian in the context of society as a whole, in addition to the individual client. This relates to social responsibility in business in terms of customer service and expectations, upholding the social regard of the profession, maintaining the social contract as the public would expect from an altruistic professional.

Veterinary ethics is a subject taught in many veterinary schools. The subject can be defined as 'a system of moral principles that apply values and judgements to the practice of veterinary medicine. Veterinary ethics combines veterinary professional ethics and the subject of animal ethics. It can be interpreted as a critical reflection on the provision of veterinary services in support of the profession's responsibilities to animal kind and mankind' (Whiting and May, 2012).

Box 5.3

RCVS Day One Competences relating to business ethics

A1.4 Be aware of the ethical responsibilities of the veterinary surgeon in relation to individual patient care and client relations, and also more generally in the community in relation to their possible impact on the environment and society as a whole.

A1.5 Be aware of the economic and emotional climate in which the veterinary surgeon operates, and respond appropriately to the influence of such pressures.

A1.7 Have an elementary knowledge of the organization and management of a veterinary practice, including:

- Awareness of own and employer's responsibilities in relation to employment and health and safety legislation, and the position relating to lay staff and public liability.

- Awareness of how fees are calculated and invoices drawn up, and the importance of following the practice's systems for record keeping and bookkeeping, including computer records and case reports.

- Ability to use information technology effectively to communicate, share, collect, manipulate and analyse information.

- Importance of complying with professional standards and policies of the practice.

A1.12 Be aware of personal limitations, and demonstrate awareness of when and from where to seek professional advice, assistance and support.

Commentary: This last item is considered to be one of the most important, and should guide all new veterinary graduates when undertaking their professional duties. Veterinary surgeons undertaking procedures on patients must at all stages in their careers be fully competent in their performance, or be under the close supervision of those who are competent. When in doubt, the new veterinary graduate must seek professional support and in the interests of animal and human health should not attempt to undertake complex procedures unsupervised.

The role of veterinary business in the profession's responsibility to each other, animals and clients is fundamental (Legood, 2000). As an academic discipline it is less developed than the analogous discipline of medical ethics; while elements may be transferable, in relation to professional conduct for example, much of the material is not directly transferable to the veterinary context due to the distinct difference in the moral status of humans and animals.

Individual veterinarians must maintain their professional duty to the client and to the animal. The Veterinary Surgeons Act (1881) gave veterinarians alone the power to practise on animals with the proviso that practice was to serve the interests of society (May, 2011; Pattison, 1984). May (2011) explains that a major difference between medical and veterinary medical professional responsibility is the expansion of the clinician–patient relationship to a triangular clinician–patient–client one. Within this clinician–patient–client relationship, the veterinary professional has duties to fulfil: first, as a veterinarian, second, as an employee and, third, to the client/animal owner.

While the primary consideration of veterinarians will always be the health and welfare of the animal under their care (RCVS, 2012a), this can be confounded by pressures of clients' personal wishes and business stressors of profit and case numbers. The economic constraints and business demands on the tripartite relationship can be a significant cause of personal stress for veterinarians.

The challenge: managing the tensions in the tripartite relationship

In practice, a potential discrepancy may begin to arise should one aspect of this tripartite relationship be compromised to favour a financial decision from the business perspective. Anecdotally, this seems to be a key concern of undergraduates who perceive that 'business' is concerned with maximizing profit and runs counter to their desire to treat animals according to the animals' best interests. They fear undue pressure from employers to run unnecessary and expensive tests or to push products that can generate profit for the practice. These concerns may emanate from negative publicity surrounding the veterinary profession in recent years, generated by disciplinary cases and investigative documentaries (e.g. BBC, 2010) highlighting cases involving poor or unethical practice. Box 5.4 contains key points from

Box 5.4

Excerpts from the restoration hearing

3. The Committee was satisfied that [the vet] knew that the diagnostic work referred to in the second element of the charge was unnecessary and would not promote [the animal's] welfare but nevertheless recommended it to [the client]. It described these procedures as intrusive and risky for [the animal].

4. The Committee found that this conduct amounted to disgraceful conduct in a professional respect. Its findings of dishonesty were, it said, very serious. [The vet] had embarked on a dishonest course of conduct, leading to his clients being misled over a number of days, and did so with a view to financial gain. He had abused his position as a veterinary surgeon.

5. In concluding that the protection of the public and upholding the reputation of the profession required that [the vet's] name be removed from the Register, that Committee expressed the view ... that honesty and trust go to the heart of professionalism and that [the vet], in betraying the trust of [the animal's] owners as he did, brought his profession into disrepute and jeopardized the welfare of an animal entrusted to his care.

attachment to their animal by offering all possible treatments to them. Nor should they overwhelm clients by outlining all the potential options and leaving them to make their decision, since clients, likely to be in a highly emotional state, may not be able to make clear informed choices. On the other hand, veterinarians should not be paternalistic, offering only those treatments that they think the client can afford in an attempt to avoid burdening them with guilt at being unable to afford life-sustaining treatments. A balance has to be struck between these extremes. It can be difficult to know how to persuade the client to do what is the best for the animal, and ethical debate surrounds the issue as to whether 'persuading' is actually part of the role of the veterinarian at all (Mullan, 2011). It is not the veterinarian's place to judge how clients may best spend their money; advocacy on the part of the animal and recommendation of the treatment which best suits the client's and animal's need is paramount: '[s]elf interests, such as practice profitability and academic interest, that could influence one recommendation above another should be recognized and put to one side' (Main, 2010). This can be a difficult balance for new graduate veterinarians to achieve. Handling difficult situations with clients can be a stressful part of working life in practice.

Operating within realms of professional competence (A1.12)

Knowing what can be achieved in general practice and what should ideally be undertaken at a referral centre can be difficult for new veterinarians. Those keen to develop their skills may be tempted to undertake work that should be undertaken by more experienced veterinarians or referred on to specialists; others lacking confidence and possibly nervous at the prospect of litigation may always opt to refer cases and unduly limit their own practice and development. Both these scenarios can cause tensions between inexperienced surgeons and their practice. The RCVS outlines the importance of making a client aware of referral options for their animals while the veterinarian in charge of the case remains within their area of competence. However, this does not mean that cases beyond the skill set of the inexperienced primary veterinarian cannot be managed with co-supervision from their more experienced colleagues, to allow for both the animal to be treated appropriately and the inexperienced colleague to gain

a recent disciplinary hearing at the RCVS where the respondent was criticized for prioritizing profit over animal welfare (RCVS DC, 2011a).

It is contended herein that good business practice is ethical business practice, which results in a motivated veterinary practice team, enhanced animal welfare and a profitable veterinary business. As an example, a practice advertising vaccinations, flea and wormer treatments and mailing reminders to customers will not only benefit from increased product sales and customer loyalty, but will also contribute to enhanced animal welfare as they remind clients of their duties as responsible pet owners.

The economic and emotional climate (A1.5)

Being 'aware of the economic and emotional climate' draws upon the veterinarian's empathy, emotional intelligence and interpersonal skills and is highly important in healthcare. On the one hand, veterinarians should not take advantage of a client's emotional experience, so long as informed consent is obtained. Any request from a client for referral, however, must be met with information to facilitate the process (RCVS, 2012c) (1.1). A recent disciplinary case of a primary veterinarian highlighted the importance of staying within achieved clinical competence; the case was supported on appeal by the Privy Council. The Committee emphasized the aggravating factors of the respondent's actions as follows: unable to refer to CPD, peer-reviewed material or accepted practice in formulation of clinical policies and being unable to appreciate that his policies were radically different from the accepted norms. The predominant reason for the removal from the register was that animal welfare and public confidence in the profession were harmed, and this was exemplified through his *'lack of appreciation of when a case was outwith his competence ... in the face of its repeated failure and the patient's continued deterioration'* and his *'lack of willingness to accept that others in the profession might know more than he, and reluctance to consider referral as an option'* (RCVS DC, 2011b).

Additionally, referring veterinarians must ensure that clients are fully informed of the level of expertise of the veterinarian to whom they are being referred and their level of qualification, i.e. 'RCVS/European/American Recognized Specialists or certificate holders' (RCVS, 2012c)(1.4). Ultimately, the veterinarian is individually responsible never to 'undertake complex procedures with which they are unfamiliar unsupervised' (RCVS, 2006, Section A2.12).

There are major professional and animal welfare ramifications if employees undertake work outside their competence. In not doing work, however, that is within their area of competence, even if that necessitates supervision, then the practice loses money as business is directed elsewhere. This can be an area of concern and conflict, especially if veterinarians feel they are being encouraged to undertake procedures by a manager motivated by either profit or an opportunity to perform a certain procedure. This is one area where ethical perspectives and clinical decisions may differ.

A1.7 Knowledge of the organization and management of a veterinary practice

Employers do not expect new veterinary graduates to be strategic business leaders. They do, however, expect a basic level of awareness that the veterinary

practice is a business. Veterinary practices operate with significant overheads and they need to generate enough income to keep the practice operational and staff in employment. A minimum requirement for new employees in any business is to be aware of pricing policies and to apply those.

Fees, pricing and record-keeping

Lowe (2009) called for the inclusion of business planning, marketing, human resource management and an awareness of the veterinary business environment to be provided to undergraduates to enable them to offer clients treatments and prevention strategies that are both cost-effective and aligned with the needs of the individual veterinary business within which they would be working (Lowe, 2009, p. 55).

New graduates are likely to require more time for individual consultations and in performing procedures. This is expected by employers, with fewer appointments being scheduled for new graduates per hour than for more experienced assistants. New veterinarians are often acutely aware that they have much to learn in order to be 'a good vet'. A lack of confidence and practical experience can mean that graduates find it difficult to charge a client for their time or they may be tempted to provide treatment, consultations or other products at no cost, to lessen what looks like an expensive bill. In a veterinary practice facing difficult economic circumstances, such behaviours can have a major impact on profitability and sustainability. Many practices have computerized systems to assist with invoicing and appropriate charging, and new graduates need to become familiar with this system and charge appropriately for services, products and treatments provided. While a veterinary practice making a profit or loss is not an ethical issue, persistent or long-term financial losses will jeopardize business survival and can therefore impact upon a veterinarian's ability to improve animal welfare in the future. Therefore, it can be argued that effective invoicing for services and collection of money is needed to safeguard future animal welfare.

Similarly, it is important not to overcharge clients. Veterinarians should be aware that different practices in different geographical areas will be able to, and will need to, charge different prices. In an affluent area of London where clients are wealthier and rental prices much higher, the price charged for a consultation will be higher than a student may have witnessed when undertaking an extramural studies placement elsewhere in a disadvantaged, rural area where business premises were attached to the home and, consequently, overheads were much lower. In practice, it can cost between £50 and £200 per hour to run a consultation room, a fact that perhaps makes the break-even and profit implications of not charging for a 15-minute consultation more readily appreciable.

Conclusions

In an increasingly challenging business environment, veterinary practice owners are seeking employees with business acumen. Indeed, RCVS outline Day One Competence requirements for new veterinarians in relation to ethical practice, professional conduct and business-related knowledge and practices. It is clear that veterinarians must charge appropriately for their services, communicate effectively with clients and ensure they operate within their competence, either individually or under the supervision of a more experienced and suitably competent veterinarian. In the current climate, the ethical management of people and practices is increasingly important.

As this chapter has demonstrated, while individuals will have a natural management style, they may need to adopt a different style in response to circumstances or to effectively manage given individuals. In this regard, the potential for HRM tools and techniques such as employee performance appraisal, staff training and development, and remuneration packages to motivate employees to perform their work to a high standard, in line with business objectives, was discussed, as were the potentially differing ethical perspectives of employee and employer, and the possible tensions between ethics and business objectives that may arise and cause stress for veterinarians working in practice.

Ethical veterinary business management should therefore be regarded as incorporating and encouraging the ethical practice of veterinary medicine while supporting good customer service, ethical pricing, sound environmental policies and a happy, motivated team. Good practice in HRM should align with the ethical and professional responsibilities of veterinarians working in practices or, at least, minimize the potential for conflict and ensure that adequate support and guidance mechanisms are in place when conflicts do arise.

Summary

This chapter has considered key concepts of management, within the context of veterinary business and professional ethics. It introduced the four functional tasks of management: planning, leading, organizing and controlling; and discussed the main management styles: autocratic, democratic and laissez-faire. Several theories of motivation, categorized as either content (Maslow, Herzberg and McClelland) or process (Vroom's expectancy or Adams' equity) theories, were also discussed. These theories illustrate that different things motivate different people, and that motivation can change over time. An understanding of motivation theories is useful for veterinarians in identifying what motivates both themselves and their colleagues. Such understanding is especially valuable for those responsible for leading a veterinary team and improving staff performance and morale.

Review questions

1. How can a veterinary practice owner introduce employee reward systems to enhance employee motivation without jeopardizing animal welfare or encouraging poor ethical practice amongst employees?
2. Which management or leadership styles are more likely to motivate employees and create good workplace relations? What would motivate or demotivate you in a workplace?
3. What are the main tensions and challenges facing practice owners in the ethical management of veterinary practices?
4. What business awareness does a new graduate veterinarian need in order to be a competent professional employee working in practice?
5. What are the main areas where a difference in ethical perspectives can arise and cause employee stress?

References

Adams, J.S., 1965. Inequity in social exchange. Advances in Experimental Social Psychology 62, 335–343.

BBC, 2010. Panorama: It shouldn't happen at a vets. Screened 3 September 2010.

Chusmir, L.H., Parker, B., 1992. Success strivings and their relationship to affective work behaviors: gender differences. J. Soc. Psychol. 132 (1), 87–99.

Cousquer, G., 2011. Principled profit-sharing? In Pract. 33 (3), 142–143.

Fayol, H., 1949. General and Industrial Administration. Pitman, London.

Heath, T.J., 2007. Longitudinal study of veterinary students and veterinary surgeons: the first 20 years. Aust. Vet. J. 85 (7), 281–289.

Henry, C., Treanor, L., 2012. The veterinary business landscape: contemporary issues and emerging trends. In: Perez-Marin, C.C. (Ed.), Veterinary Medicine: A Bird's Eye View. InTech Publishing, Rijeka, Croatia, pp. 3–16 (accessed 11.01.13). Available: http://www.intechopen.com/books/a-bird-s-eye-view-of-veterinary-medicine/the-veterinary-business-landscape-contemporary-issues-and-emerging-trends

Henry, C., Treanor, L., Baillie, S., 2011. The challenges for female small business owners and manager: a consideration of the veterinary profession. In: Cooper, C., Burke, R. (Eds.), Human Resource Management in Small Businesses: Achieving peak performance. Edward Elgar, Cheltenham, UK, pp. 216–235.

Johnson, R., 2003. HR must embrace ethics. People Management 9 (1) http://www.peoplemanagement.co.uk/pm/articles/2003/05/8844.htm

Kirby, D., 2003. Entrepreneurship. McGraw-Hill, Maidenhead, UK.

Legood, G., 2000. Veterinary Ethics. Continuum, London.

Lowe, P., 2009. Unlocking potential: a report on veterinary expertise in food animal production. DEFRA, UK.

MacDonald, C., 2012. Business ethics. http://www.businessethics.ca/definitions/business-ethics.html

Main, D.C.J., 2010. To refer or not? In Pract. 32 (4), 171.

Marcoux, A., 2008. Business ethics. In: Zalta, E.N. (Ed.), The Stanford Encyclopedia of Philosophy, http://plato.stanford.edu/archives/fall2008/entries/ethics-business/

Maslow, A.H., 1943. A theory of human motivation. Psychol. Rev. 50, 370–396.

Maslow, A.H., 1954. Motivation and Personality. Harper & Row, New York.

May, S.A., 2011. Veterinary ethics, professionalism and society. International Conference of Veterinary and Animal Ethics. Wiley-Blackwell. London.

McClelland, D.C., 1961. The Achieving Society. Van Nostrand, New York.

McDonalds v Steel & Morris, 1997. EWHC QB 3666.

McGregor, D., 1960. The Human Side of Enterprise. McGraw-Hill, New York.

Mullan, S., 2011. Comments on the dilemma in the October issue: 'Mammary mass in an overweight dog'. In Pract. 33 (10), 559.

Pattison, I., 1984. The British Veterinary Profession 1791–1948. JA Allen, London.

RCVS, 2006. Essential Competences Required of the Veterinary Surgeon. Royal College of Veterinary Surgeons, London.

RCVS, 2007. The UK Veterinary Profession in 2006: The Findings of a Survey of the Profession Conducted by the Royal College of Veterinary surgeons. Royal College of Veterinary Surgeons, London.

RCVS, 2010. The 2010 RCVS Survey of the UK Veterinary and Veterinary Nursing Professions. Royal College of Veterinary surgeons, London.

RCVS, 2012a. Code of Professional Conduct for Veterinary Surgeons.

Royal College of Veterinary Surgeons, London.

RCVS, 2012b. Supporting guidance 17: Veterinary team and business. Code of Professional Conduct for Veterinary Surgeons. Royal College of Veterinary Surgeons, London.

RCVS, 2012c. Policy on Continuing Professional Development for Veterinary Surgeons. Royal College of Veterinary Surgeons, London.

RCVS DC, 2011a. Royal College of Veterinary Surgeons v Kfir Segev. London.

RCVS DC, 2011b. Royal College of Veterinary Surgeons v Joseph Lennox Holmes. London.

Rollinson, D., Broadfield, A., 2002. Organisational Behaviour and Analysis: an Integrated Approach, second ed. Pearson Education, Harlow, UK.

Rose, A., 2007. Ethics and human resource management. In: Porter, C., Bingham, C., Simmonds, D. (Eds.), Exploring Human Resource Management. McGraw-Hill, London, pp. 29–43.

Stahl, M.J., 1983. Achievement, power and managerial motivation: selecting managerial talent with the job choice exercise. Personnel Psychology 36 (4), 775–790.

Taylor, F.W., 1911. Principles of Scientific Management. Harper, New York.

Ulrich, D., 1996. Human Resource Champions: The Next Agenda for Adding Value and Delivering Results. Harvard Business School Press, Boston, MA.

Vroom, V., 1964. Work and Motivation. Wiley, New York.

Whiting, M., May, S., 2012. A multiple format cumulative learning structure for veterinary ethics. Presented at the American Association of Veterinary Medical Colleges Conference, Alexandria, VA.

Documenting and investigating the entrepreneurial trade in illegal veterinary medicines in the United Kingdom and Ireland

6

Robert Smith   Martin Whiting

CHAPTER OVERVIEW

Entrepreneurship has the potential to reinvigorate, and perhaps even revolutionize, the veterinary industry. However, it is not a panacea to mend all ills; it can also have a darker side, as entrepreneurship manifests itself along a spectrum from informal entrepreneurship to criminal entrepreneurship (Smith, 2009; Gottschalk, 2009). There is a moral dimension to entrepreneurship, and with regard to the veterinary industry the illegal trade in medicines is a contemporary example of criminal entrepreneurship. The illegal trade is a hidden and thus a deniable crime that occurs at the interface of veterinary business and free enterprise. This practice has hit the veterinary press headlines of late and, as such, is both a hot topic and an example of *rural criminal entrepreneurship* (Davis and Potter, 1991).

LEARNING OUTCOMES

After reading this chapter, students will be able to:
* Be aware of incidents of criminal entrepreneurship that may be present in and related to their profession.
* Demonstrate the links between legitimate veterinary business and criminal entrepreneurship.
* Identify key case examples of the negative trade in the international market, as well as the profession's response to such cases.
* Highlight the dangers to both human and animal health and welfare through the risk of using illegitimate medicines.
* Identify the areas of financial loss from the veterinary profession to the illegal trade in medicines.

Introduction

One normally associates the practice of criminal entrepreneurship with serious and organized criminal groups such as the Mafia or other organized criminal cartels (Arlacchi, 1986; Smith, 1978), not rogue farmers, stable hands, stud bosses or, more contentiously, unscrupulous veterinarians, pharmacists and others involved in the veterinary profession. This point, although contentious, is important in this chapter which spans veterinary science, entrepreneurship and criminality.

The illegal trade in medicines for use in animals is particularly damaging to the veterinary profession, as not only does it represent a source of lost revenue for the business, but, additionally, places animal health and welfare at risk. A veterinarian has a responsibility to uphold public interest in animal welfare and protect the safety of food animals; therefore, it falls to the veterinarians to be aware of, detect and report the unlawful use of medicines on animals.

The veterinary industry in the UK and Ireland: a review of the literature

This review of the literature both situates and contextualizes criminal entrepreneurship in relation to the veterinary industry in the UK and Ireland.

© 2014, Elsevier Ltd.

The stereotype of the veterinarian

First we must define what we mean by the term *veterinarian*. In the UK, the term veterinary surgeon is defined by statute (Veterinary Surgeons Act 1966). An individual becomes a veterinarian by the power invested in the President of the Royal College of Veterinary Surgeons (RCVS) through the 1966 Royal Charter. This charter enables the president to add the names of people to a statutory list of veterinarians, and only those on that list are veterinarians.[1] This emphasis on legal responsibilities is important in this chapter. This statutory protected title limits veterinarians to be the sole profession able to diagnose and treat animals.

Traditionally, veterinarians are held in high esteem, a position which is broadly in line with the notion of the rural idyll (Mingay, 1989) in which veterinarians enact and perform their everyday duties. The veterinary industry in the UK and Ireland has, traditionally, been viewed as a bastion of male domination, with men running the industry's institutions (Grant and Greaves, 2009, p. 9; Windsor, 2002). This still largely holds true in rural veterinary practice, which remains male dominated despite the changing demographic relating to the dominance of female veterinarians in urban practice (Grant and Greaves, 2009; Henry *et al.*, 2010). Indeed, Henry *et al.* (2011) question the viability of this traditional model of veterinary practice. Moreover, the veterinarian is socially constructed and viewed by the public as a kindly, stoic man.[2] More recently, the veterinarian has been constructed in popular culture and rural folklore as a hero figure, a purveyor of rural expertise (see Grant and Greaves, 2009). It is of relevance that there is a similar heroic construct in relation to farmers; indeed, for Saugeres (2002) there is a discourse in farming which embodies the inherited relationship between the farmer and the land whereby 'good farmers' possess an innate understanding of nature. A sympathetic feel for the land is often associated with traditional farming, and this intuitively stretches to the veterinary profession. Saugeres argues that, conversely, the alienated and exploitative attitude of the 'bad farmer' towards nature is associated with modern agriculture and agri-business (and by extension entrepreneurship). Similarly, for Malecki (2006) the 'lives and livelihoods' of entrepreneurs in rural contexts are embedded in their socio-economic circumstances. These factors, perhaps, explain why some farmers adopt a cynical and cunning single-minded pursuit of money. Such farmers fit the cultural stereotype of the '*bad farmer*' (Nerlich *et al.*, 2002). This notion of the 'rogue farmer' (Smith, 2004; Smith and McElwee, 2013) is of great importance to veterinary practice because it stands between the unwritten moral contract that exists between the veterinarian and the farmer as a client. Accepting that farmers are not a homogeneous breed (McElwee, 2006), and that some may breach their public trust in upholding animal welfare, or even act criminally, loosens the bond of reciprocal trust. As they go about their daily business veterinarians undoubtedly witness some acts of immoral or illegal practice committed by their clients, and it is often easy to 'turn a blind eye'. Many are, no doubt, dealt with pragmatically with sound advice and verbal warnings.

The changing landscape of the veterinary industry

The veterinary industry within the UK is mainly operated under an entrepreneurial model of private practice, with practices catering for geographical areas and veterinary specialisms. This situates the organization of the majority of veterinary practices within the framework of being a SME (small and medium size business).[3] However, Grant and Greaves (2009) also identify other types of veterinary practice in the UK, such as the category of the State Employed Veterinarians. This (re)construction of the veterinarian as an administrator, policy maker and enforcement officer (such as those employed by DEFRA in the UK) is somewhat at odds with the traditional bucolic image of rurality (see Budge *et al.*, 2008) and of the jovial country veterinarian of popular culture.

Cooper and Cooper (2008) argue that veterinarians have long played a role in the investigation of illegality

---

[1] A person needs to have an approved veterinary degree and to be a member of the RCVS. Also there are eight MsRCVS who do not require nor do they have a veterinary degree but are lawfully able to practise as veterinarians under a grandfather clause. It is a complicated area. According to Grant and Greaves (2009), '*A veterinarian is defined as a fully trained veterinary surgeon and member of the Royal College of Veterinary Surgeons (RCVS) with accompanying legal responsibilities.*' This is important as there are many recorded instances of persons falsely purporting to be veterinarians.

[2] This results from the fictional and deeply stereotypical television portrayals such as those of the British Veterinarian Alf Wright who wrote under the pseudonym James Herriot, which formed the basis of the hugely popular BBC series '*All Creatures Great and Small*'. The archetypal country veterinarian was held in esteem by the rural public, gentlemen farmers and the local squirarchy. For a discussion of the development of the industry prior to the 1960s see Wright (1961).

[3] An SME is any business with fewer than 250 employees.

that directly or indirectly involves animals, and stress that the role of the veterinarian in such instances is accelerating rapidly. Another matter arising from the state ownership of veterinary knowledge and expertise is that it changes the traditional role of veterinarians in the eyes of their traditional communities of practice, such as farming and the equine industry, because they have a formalized legal obligation to report breaches of regulation, crimes and offences. Thus they become part of the intelligence-gathering apparatus of the state. Kogan and McConnell (2001) stress that the upbringing of veterinary applicants reflects their choice of career locations, i.e. that people who grow up in urban settings tend to practise in urban settings upon qualification, and that the rural veterinary applicant tends to gravitate towards rural practice. Moreover, Grant and Greaves describe an industry that has been undergoing a number of changes, including:

- a gender shift in the composition of a profession dominated by men to one in which women make up by far the greater part of the graduate intake;
- a trend away from large-animal (i.e. farmed livestock) work to small-animal (i.e. domestic companion animals) work;
- a trend towards more multi-centre practices owned by companies with professional financial managers;
- increasing costs on veterinary services.

These industry pressures are important in the context of this chapter because they highlight a move away from the traditional image of the veterinarian towards a more businesslike, entrepreneurial approach where finance – not merely expertise – becomes an important influence and concern. Even if veterinarians shun the entrepreneurial persona, their competitors may not, and an awareness of the entrepreneurial nature of veterinary business becomes as essential as veterinary knowledge itself. This leads us to consider how criminal entrepreneurship is manifested and could damage the veterinary industry.

Contextualizing criminal entrepreneurship and the veterinary industry

As a practice, entrepreneurship is associated with traits such as risk-taking behaviour (Brockhaus, 1980). In the case of the veterinary industry one has to differentiate between the label and the behaviour

because veterinary medicine is regarded as a profession gained after many years of academic study and practical experience; one cannot become a veterinarian without being accredited. Thus, unlike other areas of business one cannot simply become a veterinary entrepreneur, albeit one does not need to be a veterinarian to start a practice. The owner of a practice does not need to be a vet; for example, the large chain of (currently) 232 veterinary practices, six veterinary laboratories and one crematorium managed by the overarching company CVS is mainly managed by non-veterinarians (CVS, 2012).[4] It is thus a partially restricted occupation in terms of entrepreneurial opportunity. This does not mean that individual veterinarians cannot learn to be entrepreneurial and adopt entrepreneurial ideologies and practices. This is a particularly salient point because entrepreneurship is about change, and change often occurs slowly. It is also of relevance that examples of what constitutes entrepreneurship are often industry specific. (For an overview of entrepreneurship in the agricultural sector see studies by Alsos et al., 2011; Iaquinto and Spinelli, 2006; McElwee, 2006; and Sharma et al., 2010.)

Existing writings on criminal entrepreneurship (such as Hobbs, 1988) are location and sector specific and have a tendency towards descriptiveness. The most useful definition is that of Baumol (1990, p. 14), who defines criminal entrepreneurship as 'the imaginative pursuit of position, with limited concern about the means used to achieve the purpose'. In the criminological literature there is an assumption that rural crime is committed by marauding urban criminals, and that the indigenous population are always the victims (Dingwall and Moody, 1999; Smith, 2010). This chapter challenges this assumption, demonstrating that examples of criminal entrepreneurship can come from within the industry.

The illegal veterinary drugs trade

The illegal trade in veterinary medicines is the illegal sale, purchase and distribution of medicine that is then used on animals with or without the authorization of a veterinarian. Any medicine given to animals to diagnose or treat a disease must be done under the

---

[4] The names of the directors and management personnel advertised by CVS were cross-referenced with the RCVS register of veterinary surgeons (CVS Personnel 2012). Available: http://www.cvsukltd.co.uk/personnel.htm [accessed 19 September 2012]

authority of a veterinarian, and animal owners who self-treat their animals may be in breach of this.

The trade consists of several subsets of practice, as follows:

- the *'parallel trade in the pharmaceutical industry'* whereby legally manufactured drugs are sold at a price difference between countries resulting in labelling, etc., not matching the standards of the country into which they are imported (Barfield and Groombridge, 1999; Kanavos and Costa-Font, 2005);
- legally manufactured drugs which have reached their recommended expiry date (Daughton and Ternes, 1999) and are offloaded elsewhere;
- the fraudulent sale of one type of banned drug as another;
- legally manufactured drugs which have been stolen;
- the counterfeit trade whereby the drugs are manufactured illegally by chemists for an organized criminal conspiracy (Liang, 2005; Stearn, 2004).

Although this chapter is primarily concerned with the illegal UK trade in unauthorized veterinary medicines, it is obviously a global problem involving both unauthorized and counterfeit veterinary products.[5] This gives an indication of the potential illegal revenues to be had by unscrupulous operators. It is a subject which the pharmaceutical industry takes very seriously. (For further information on the counterfeit trade see the Bayer website entry on the subject. For a wider discussion of the counterfeit trade in veterinary medicines see work by Stearn, 2004, and Terzić et al., 2011). According to Terzić et al. (2011), 10% of all medicinal products on the market are counterfeit. Although the majority of those medicinal products are intended for use in human medicine, numbers of those used in veterinary medicine are on the rise. Although it is difficult to assess the extent of the illegal trade, the examples discussed in this chapter provide evidence that it is a pernicious and very real problem. The key case study included in this chapter is the company Eurovet, which had thousands of customers and a multi-million-pound enterprise. This case example should act as a warning signal to veterinarians and to the authorities as to the potential scale of the problem.

Methodology and the development of an investigative mindset

The primary methodology in the study presented in this chapter is that of documentary research (see Mogalakwe, 2006; Platt, 1981; Scott, 1990, 2006). This methodology is essential to this inquiry because much of what we know about the illegal trade in veterinary medicines comes to us from the media and, in particular, newspapers. Mogalakwe (2006) lists one of the strengths of documentary research as being that it allows one to access 'difficult to reach' research topics. Given that in using documentary research one is reliant upon what is reported by journalists, it is vital that we as academics take care to *'read between the lines'* (Fitzgerald, 2007) to reach a more nuanced understanding of the issues involved. Furthermore, newspaper and media articles are useful in developing objective case studies (Yin, 2003), as reported below. For this chapter, this particular approach led to the development of the micro case stories illustrating examples from two geographical contexts: namely Britain and Ireland. Such examples are necessary as they serve to document the trade in illegal veterinary medicines.

It is also necessary to desensationalize the cases and recontextualize them in relation to entrepreneurship in order to build a rudimentary profile of the typical trader in illegal veterinary products by taking cognisance of some of the shared commonalities and features of the cases. In criminological circles, profiling is an accepted investigatory practice, albeit the mapping exercise for this chapter stops short of being a full profiling exercise, given the small number of traders involved in the high-profile prosecutions discussed below. From this it is possible to conceptualize and develop typologies as further cases and prosecutions emerge in the coming years. The cases are presented below.

Geographical context 1: the Irish connection

There is a well-documented Irish connection to the trade, with Eire being suspected of being a source of such illegal medicines.[6] In 2004, Medicines

---

[5] Sourced at http://www.fao.org/news/story/en/item/123165/icode/. According to the International Federation of Animal Health (IFAH), the value of the official market for veterinary drugs in Africa alone is around $400 million a year.

[6] This case study was developed from entries from the website http://www.dhsspsni.gov.uk/index/pas/pas-enforcementaction-pressreleases.htm and, as such, the material is already in the public domain. All the cases discussed are from the website.

Enforcement Officers from the Department of Health, Social Services and Public Safety (DHSSPS) interdicted a major operation to manufacture illegal veterinary drugs. After a prolonged multi-agency investigation they seized a large quantity of unauthorized and counterfeit veterinary medicines from locations across Northern Ireland and the Republic.[7] In 2005, a large quantity of illegal veterinary medicines were found abandoned at a rural location on waste ground. In 2007, a veterinary practitioner was convicted and given a conditional discharge at Londonderry Magistrates Court for 12 charges relating to the possession of illegal veterinary medicines. Again in 2008, following the seizure of unlicensed veterinary medicines, a County Down veterinary surgeon was formally advised by the RCVS to comply with all relevant legislation including Veterinary Medicines legislation – the Veterinary Medicinal Products Directive 2001/82/EC (as amended).[8] This aspect of the case is fascinating because it suggests that some veterinarians may be involved in the trade, and further highlights that it is not just an example of predatory criminal behaviour by outsiders. In June 2009, at Belfast Crown Court a man was sentenced to six months' imprisonment, suspended for two years after having been caught in possession of illegal veterinary medicines and supplying counterfeit veterinary products. As a result of a multi-agency investigation[9] in May 2011, two brothers from the Lurgan area were each fined £750.00 plus court costs, having pleaded guilty to charges of unlawfully importing, possessing and exporting unauthorized veterinary medicines. The brothers had been caught in possession of a large quantity of unauthorized veterinary medicines, including antibiotics and steroids primarily intended for the greyhound and equine market. A large

amount of cash in sterling and euros was also recovered following searches of residential properties in the Lurgan area. The brothers had sourced the medicines in Australia and were distributing them in Northern Ireland and Eire. The activities of the brothers indicate an evident entrepreneurial flair in that they were acting as importers of the drugs linking various networks together. This example further evidences the multinational nature of the crime. In November 2011, an agricultural merchant from Fermanagh was also fined £2000 for possession and supply of prescription-only veterinary medicines without proper qualification. In November 2011, a haul of drugs, worth several thousand pounds and including veterinary antibiotics and other veterinary medicines intended for the treatment of large numbers of farm animals, was recovered from a residential property in Ballymena after another multi-agency operation.

The issue is also obviously a pharmaceutical industry problem. In 2005, the Statutory Committee of the Pharmaceutical Society for Northern Ireland issued a reprimand to a pharmacist for selling veterinary products other than by a prescription under the Medicines Act 1968, section 58(2). In 2007, another pharmacist was convicted at Newry Magistrates Court on charges of possession of unauthorized veterinary medicines in contravention of the Veterinary Medicines Regulations 2005. In 2009, an industrial chemist was sentenced to six months' imprisonment, suspended for two years, after pleading guilty to charges relating to the placing on the market and supply of unauthorized veterinary medicines. He also pleaded guilty to the supply of a counterfeit veterinary product.

This geographically situated micro case study is of interest because, although it does not provide proof of a conspiracy or link the separate accused together, it does highlight the involvement of veterinarians, criminal entrepreneurs, an agricultural merchant, farmers and pharmacists and evidences that it is a continuing criminal enterprise.

[7] Involving PSNI, Garda Siochana, Department of Agriculture and Rural Development and the Department of Agriculture and Food, in the Republic of Ireland.

[8] The Veterinary Medicinal Products Directive 2001/82/EC (as amended) sets out the controls on the manufacture, authorization, marketing, distribution and post-authorization surveillance of veterinary medicines applicable in all European member states. The Directive provides the basis for the UK controls on veterinary medicines, which are set out nationally in the Veterinary Medicines Regulations. The Regulations are revoked and replaced on an annual basis after consultation with interested groups to ensure that they are up to date and fit for purpose. See the website http://www.vmd.defra.gov.uk/public/vmr.aspx.html for further details.

[9] Involving the Department of Health, Social Services and Public Safety (DHSSPS) Medicines Regulatory Group, the Department of Agriculture and Rural Development (DARD), the PSNI and regulatory counterparts from ROI.

Geographical context 2: the Eurovet case

This case study relates to the well-publicized Eurovet case.[10] Regine (nee Langley) and Ronald Meddes, the Picardy-based British owners of a company trading

[10] This case study was based on a reading of 11 newspaper and magazine articles listed in the documentary evidence section.

under the name of Eurovet, are described in the press as running a 'black market empire'.[11] The illegal operation run by the Meddes was described by the judge as an industrial-scale operation. The illegal drugs they supplied included anti-inflammatories, anabolic steroids, tranquillizers, antibiotics, sedatives, painkillers and other miscellaneous products administered to horses, household pets and farm animals. The business had all the appearances and trappings of a legitimate small business – for example, many of the medicines were sold to UK customers by telephone, fax and online. This was no 'back street' or 'under the counter' illicit trade conducted in pubs or out of the boot of a vehicle in a car park. In fact, it was computer accounts and customer details from the business which exposed the scale of the illegal enterprise. The turnover between January 2004 and May 2007 was allegedly £5.6 million. The scam is said to have netted the couple between £6 million and £13.5 million. Their trade in unauthorized and prescription-only medicines is said to have reached more than 4000 British customers from properties in France and warehouses in Belgium and Kent.

The case was sparked off in 2006 when DEFRA Investigation Services began investigating on behalf of the VMD when a small seizure of illegal medicines occurred. This led to other investigations, which all linked back to a single source. Follow-up inquiries led to further, larger seizures at premises in Ashford, Dover, Aldershot and at Stansted Airport. In May 2007, the VMD contacted the French authorities, who seized in excess of 20 tonnes of illegal medicines. Unperturbed by the illegality, the couple quickly relocated the business to Belgium. A further raid in 2008 shut this operation down, but inquiries established that the illegal trade actually continued during 2009 and 2010 via a company registered in Hungary.

Regine and Ronald Meddes are credited with flooding the UK market with unlawful veterinary drugs. They are described, respectively, as being a stud farm boss and a riding school owner. They are further credited with playing a key role in organizing the £6 million scam, said to be the biggest of its kind in Europe. Ronald Meddes was described in the press as having a 'colourful past' – a disgraced ex-Lloyd's trader and convicted fraudster. This last point is important in terms of establishing a past entrepreneurial provenance and to the issue of entrepreneurial pluriactivity as a capital accumulation strategy (De Silva and Kodithuwakku, 2011). Meddes and Langley were well known in equestrian circles. The business initially evaded compliance with EU regulations by purporting to trade for the Russian export market. The scale of their illicit operation can be gauged from the evidence that some of their veterinary medicines enjoyed the largest market share in the UK, outselling legitimate products; indeed, just one of their many delivery companies transported 8.5 tonnes of black-market drugs into the UK over a two-year period. Additionally, there was a threefold price mark-up on medicines brought in from India. Investigators discovered paperwork documenting total sales of £13.5 million over a six-year period.

The Meddes were sentenced to 20 and 28 months' jail at Croydon Crown Court on 7 July 2011. Eleven others from the UK and France have been sentenced for their part in a £6 million black-market veterinary medicines scheme. It is of note that these included a management consultant and his wife who owned a stud farm; a haulage contractor who acted as a distributor in the UK; an artificial insemination practitioner; an accountant; a bookkeeper; two farmers; a secretary; a driver; and a pensioner. The consultant apparently received half-tonne deliveries of medication at a time from the French company, and was accused of buying £155 000 of veterinary medicines between January 2004 and September 2008. There was a 25% mark-up on medicines sold to the farmers. The accountant, who set up the company and a bank account, also admitted money laundering. The pensioner had a colourful history, having been convicted in 2006 of similar offences and of having falsely purported to be a veterinarian. He was apparently well known in equestrian circles for selling fake medicines out of the boot of a vehicle at horse fairs.

Steve Dean, Chief Executive of the Government's Veterinary Medicines Directorate (VMD), which prosecuted the case, said: *'This was a significant commercial enterprise which seriously attacked the principle of safe and effective veterinary medicines.'*

---

[11] They were ironically nicknamed Ronnie and Reggie by the press. The sobriquet Ronnie and Reggie was made infamous by the notorious London gangsters, the Kray twins. Equally ironically, a perusal of the press images of both Meddes and Lansley shows a successful middle-aged couple who look like 'the couple next door'. Between January 2004 and November 2010, the couple ran a series of businesses under the 'Eurovet' banner, including: ZAO Eurovet International; Euro Exports CIS Ltd; Global Animal Pharmaceuticals; and the Animal Pharmacy. It should be noted that company has no connection to the legitimate and established business Eurovet Animal Health Ltd of Cambridge. The use of deliberately confusing trade names is a feature of organized criminality and is used to confuse investigators. See author unattributed (2011b–2011 h).

The trial judge even commented upon the entrepreneurial nature of the illegal venture and commented: *'You could not resist trying to make money from this trade, you found a niche in the market and you exploited it.'* It is also significant that the warehouse housed offices and a team of migrant workers because it appears that the latter-day 'Ronnie and Reggie' exploited Eastern European workers to reduce the costs of the business. An investigation is under way in relation to the Proceeds of Crime Act to recover the assets of the individuals involved.

This geographically situated micro case study is of interest because it provides proof of a conspiracy of industry insiders all linked through Eurovet as a criminal enterprise. Given the occupations and professions listed above for Meddes and for the other accused in both geographically confined cases, it is easy to position them as entrepreneurs or at least in engaging in entrepreneurial behaviour because they created value for themselves and extracted the equivalent monetary value between the price differential for the illegal drugs.

However, Sarasvathy's (2001) *'theory of effectuation'* provides a much better explanation of their entrepreneurial activities. Sarasvathy (2001) argues that entrepreneurs start their venture with three types of 'means' (as opposed to capital). They know who they are, what they know and whom they know. Using these means they exploit the contingencies open to them in their own particular circumstances. Meddes used his entrepreneurial social capital, his prior experience in business and his contacts (old and new) to set up an online veterinary medicines business. As suggested by Baumol's definition, he does not particularly appear to have concerned himself with the legality of the venture. He and his associates were guilty of practising criminal entrepreneurship. Sarasvathy's theory is more convincing than trying to guess whether he was pushed or pulled into entrepreneurship. Criminal entrepreneurs practise their own form of entrepreneurship because they can. Baumol accepts that even ostensibly moral entrepreneurs may lead a parasitical existence that damages the economy, and that the concept of entrepreneurial reward lies at the heart of stimulating entrepreneurial activity because eventually a pay-off is sought. It is also of relevance that Sarasvathy (2001, p. 262), mirroring Baumol's definition, considers the entrepreneur to be an *'imaginative actor who seizes contingent opportunities and exploits any and all means at hand to fulfil a plurality of current and future aspirations'*.

Profiling the typical offender

The profile of the accused in the micro case studies is far removed from buying illegal medicines in a public house or from the back of a van. These cases highlight that the trade in illegal veterinary medicines is no 'back street' operation run by members of the criminal fraternity. What is surprising about the profile of those involved in this illegal trade is how they do not fit the archetypal profile of the stereotypical urban criminal, as the following points illustrate:

1. The key players have established entrepreneurial identities and occupations. In this respect it is tempting to consider them as rural examples of white-collar criminality (Gottschalk and Smith, 2011; Green, 2006; Sutherland, 1949).

2. Many were known in their local communities and communities of practice as the epitome of respectability. The press coverage of the saga highlighted the celebrity nature, and emphasis was placed on the fact that they lived in a *'secluded 11-bedroom farm house'*.

3. Many were late middle aged or elderly, with one being described as a pensioner. This is perhaps relevant for developing an investigative strategy in that it is consistent with the ageing profile of the farming community.

The attitude of some farmers to the illegal trade is telling. Comments located by the authors on an Internet blog site[12] relating to the veterinary scandal are interesting and include allegations that veterinarians routinely charge farmers extortionate, inflationary prices for medicines. There is talk of 'monopolies', 'cartels' and of sympathy for black marketers, as well as accusations of professional protectionism and restrictive bureaucracy. Collectively, the comments highlight the condoning of sourcing alternative cheaper medicines, even if they are sourced illegally, and a call for a fairer pricing system for medicines. These comments suggest that there is a problem, and lay the blame on the side of the veterinary industry, politicians and bureaucrats and not on the side of the criminal entrepreneurs who operate the illegal trade. It is significant that none of the bloggers blames the pharmaceutical industry or those whom Hoffman *et al.* (2011) refer to as *'pharmaceutical entrepreneurs'*. The National Farmers Union vice president Gwyn Jones

---

[12] Available: http://www.farmersguardian.com/home/livestock/livestock-news/13-convicted-for-%C2%A36m-veterinarian-medicine-smuggling/40167.article.

has called for a simplified veterinary medicines market to allow farmers better access to products at lower prices, arguing that *'divergent laws for the approval and registration of products across Europe were making it difficult for farmers to access vital medicines'*. Jones further argued that different rules across the EU add a level of complexity which can push the price up, and that there is little transparency in the regulatory procedure (Author unattributed, 2011a). The Eurovet scandal is a classic example of how the entrepreneurially minded undercut existing provision and created a market for their services, and should serve as a warning to the industry. Granted, the scheme was criminal, but then not all entrepreneurs practise productive entrepreneurship (Baumol, 1990). It is also of interest that Baumol (1990) argued that policies impeding moral entrepreneurship (such as pricing policies) can cause entrepreneurs to switch to less productive, less ethical methods.

It is also of relevance that government veterinarians often highlight the public health angle to the trade as opposed to the organized nature of the criminality involved. For example, after the Eurovet case, Steve Dean (of the VMD) stressed that *'Incorrect use of medication of unknown origin and dubious* [sic. unknown] *quality compromises animal health and welfare, increases the risk of harmful residues in the food chain and* [sic. potentially] *raises the spectre of unnecessary antibiotic resistance'*. A clearer message might have been sent to the public had the case been dealt with by the Serious and Organized Crime Agency (SOCA).

Tannenbaum (1995) argues that although veterinary ethics is a major challenge facing the profession today, there is little literature on the subject, and very little serious work is conducted on ethics in veterinary schools. According to Tannenbaum, veterinarians are said to serve two masters – animal patients and human clients – and often there is a conflict of interest. An additional third master of a profitable business model should be included in Tannenbaum's list. As has been demonstrated in this chapter, increasingly veterinarians have a moral and legal obligation to the organs of the state. Grant and Greaves (2009, p. 36) argue that there are different constructions of veterinary expertise, and it is apparent that there is scope within the State Veterinary Service (SVS) for the employment of forensic veterinary specialists (Brown, 2009; Cooper and Cooper, 2008) with the necessary knowledge to investigate and interdict those who engage in the illegal trade in veterinary drugs and

other farm/industry-based crime.[13] How then can these case studies be used to help veterinary practitioners and law enforcement officials investigate the crime and criminal practices described above? It is to this issue that we now turn and, in particular, to the role of veterinarians in investigating criminal practices.

Investigating the crime and criminal practices

It is difficult to investigate illegal trading in veterinary medicines because one must establish if it is actually an illegal drug that is being traded. Alternatively, it could be a counterfeit drug, or a generic drug that is infringing on copyright, or an authentic branded drug illegally imported, or a counterfeit legally imported. Furthermore, it could relate to a drug being used incorrectly by the client off-licence, or perhaps a correct drug used in the correct way for a disease but used without a veterinarian. There are many elements to illegal drug use in animals that are highly veterinary specific. The laws which govern the illegal trade are:

- the Marketing Authorisations for Veterinary Medicinal Products Regulations 1994, as imposed by Sections 108–110 of the Medicines Act 1968, as appropriate;
- the Veterinary Medicines Regulations 2011 (as amended).

The problem with using illegally manufactured veterinary products is that they may contain unauthorized antibiotics or other compounds which, when introduced indiscriminately into the food chain, can be harmful to human health.[14] The crime of trading in illegal veterinary drugs is difficult to detect and interdict primarily because it occurs in a private business domain into which the practising veterinarian, and indeed law enforcement officials, have limited access. The Eurovet case was focused mainly on illegal trading in veterinary drugs and not upon the issue of trading in illegal veterinary drugs. The two crimes, although similar, have substantially different effects on animal welfare which are of primary concern to the veterinary reader in that the

---

[13] Forensic veterinary medicine is of increasing importance. Legal and other cases in which a veterinary input is likely to be required include those relating to unexpected death of animals, welfare, abuse and breaches of conservation law.

[14] Sourced from http://www.ergogenics.org/farmdrugs.html.

former crime does not have the same concern in relation to introducing health risks as the latter. Moreover, many of the drugs, irrespective of the category, are sold via telephone, fax and online, so the chances of patrolling police officers or other law enforcement officials stumbling upon the crime are rare. This imbues the transactions with the appearance of legal authenticity. As with so many investigations into organized crime, the authorities are reliant upon information from the public and from informants. Investigating the illegal practice first of all entails acknowledging its existence, and thereafter identifying key players such as those discussed above in the case studies. Veterinarians and others involved in the industry are required to be more vigilant and to report such suspicions.

An identified problem with investigating rural criminality is that often there are multiple agencies involved, with incompatible intelligence databases (Smith, 2010), and each agency has a small part of the picture. There is also a perception of rural Omertà[15] or 'code of silence' not to interfere with illegal activities, which Barclay *et al.* (2004) refer to as the darker side of rural Gemeinschaft (community). Barclay *et al.* argued that in particular rural communities there is an aversion to sharing information with the authorities, and that some criminal practices become an open secret to all but the law enforcement community. To return to the argument articulated above, the archetypal jovial country veterinarian is seen as the farmers' friend, and quite often this may necessitate cultivating a working relationship. Changing the veterinary mindset into an investigative one is difficult.

This brings the issue of deviant behaviour amongst veterinary practitioners into play; this is not a novel concept (see, for example, Gauthier, 2001). According to Gauthier, veterinarians use neutralization techniques to counteract ethically or legally problematic lapses in the performance of their professional duties. Although set in an American context, the study demonstrates that although (by and large) veterinarians are honest, they sometimes question the validity of rules in relation to their roles in certain circumstances. Through the use of neutralization techniques, veterinarians facilitate behaviours that outsiders to

their circumstances might question on legal or ethical grounds – such as turning a blind eye to some questionable rural practices which others consider unethical. For some veterinarians there is a dilemma between educating out bad practice and enforcing legal sanctions (Gottschalk and Smith, 2011).

The issue of veterinary ethics is also relevant here (Hannah, 2002), as is the issue of professional behaviour of veterinarians. In the UK, the 'RCVS Code of Professional Conduct for Veterinary Surgeons' (RCVS, 2012) governs and guides how veterinarians should conduct themselves. The Code recognizes that, on occasions, the professional responsibilities in the Code may conflict with each other and veterinary surgeons may be presented with a dilemma. The Code stresses that in such situations veterinary surgeons should always resolve the conflict having regard first to animal welfare. It is significant that veterinarians' first responsibility is towards the care of animals. They are advised to fulfil their professional responsibilities, by maintaining five principles of practice:

- professional competence;
- honesty and integrity;
- independence and impartiality;
- client confidentiality and trust;
- professional accountability.

The only advice in relation to the illegal trade in veterinary medicines appears to be that veterinary surgeons who prescribe, supply and administer medicines must do so responsibly.

The illegal trade in veterinary medicines can and does impact upon veterinary business in terms of lost revenue to the industry at a time when it can least afford it. The first question which one must ask is '*How can my practice arrange its business enterprise so as to protect itself and its clients against illegal trade?*' There are no easy answers, but awareness is the first step. Henry and Treanor (2012) suggest that changing business practices, such as the increase in online sales of veterinary medicines, may also have impacted on the changing veterinary landscape. This creates a squeeze on veterinary practices' profit margins, and consequentially there is a need to revise pricing structures for core veterinary services (Henry and Treanor, 2012). It is clear that clients will seek the best financial deal for the care of their animals, and in the current economic climate this is accentuated. In certain respects a veterinary practice will have a monopoly over its clients in their ability to freely purchase drugs (for example, a client may

---

[15] The Italian concept of Omertà is a popular cultural attitude or code of honour that places heavy importance on a deep-rooted 'code of silence', non-cooperation with authorities, and non-interference in the illegal (and legal) actions of others. The concept is recognized to be one of the universal problems facing investigators of rural criminality (see, for example, Smith, 2010).

not supply their own anaesthetic drugs or vaccinations for the veterinarian to use on their own animals). However, the client does have freedom to obtain other medicines (for example, tablet-form antibiotics, analgesics or flea and worm treatment) for their animals via a prescription if they wish. This allows clients to 'shop' for the best price they can obtain for their medicines, but denial of this freedom to clients, or the disproportionate cost of drugs from a practice compared to other pharmacies, may push clients to obtain their medicines from alternative and, potentially unknowingly, illegitimate sources. The Eurovet case demonstrates a substantial market of £6 million to £13.5 million that was lost from the veterinary profession in terms of drug sales, with an additional risk to the client, and subsequently to their animals, that the drugs may be fraudulent. Thus, in order to uphold veterinarians' declaration to place animal welfare above all else, appropriate business modelling should incorporate a pricing scheme that is competitive to online pharmacies and a system of making clients aware of the potential risks from illegitimate online businesses.

There are a number of potential routes for practices to detect and combat this illegal trade if necessary. The obvious route is to arrange awareness and training seminars where experienced colleagues can pass on the investigatory tricks of the trade. For example, all veterinary medicinal products in the UK must be authorized.[16] The official body responsible for marketing authorizations is the Veterinary Medicines Directorate. All products have a VM number on their label; if a bottle does not have a VM label it is likely to be an unauthorized counterfeit product. Products with a marketing authorization are given unique numbers, preceded by the letters 'VM'; therefore, if a product does not have a VM number on its label, it has not been authorized. A VM issued in respect of a legitimate product provides assurance to consumers of the product's safety, quality and efficacy.

Act responsibly – only buy veterinary medicines from reputable sources. Look out for counterfeit labels, large quantities of bottles for injectable products and large quantities of raw materials used in the manufacture of veterinary drugs. Hack (2011) stresses that the veterinary profession can play an important role in combating the illegal trade in the use of veterinary medicines by being vigilant and reporting

any suspicions to the VMD. Dean (2009) argues that many of the illegal veterinary medicines are bought from abroad via the internet. According to Terzić et al. (2011), suppressing the production, distribution and use of counterfeit medicinal products requires sound and constant cooperation of inspection services, manufacturers and distributors, drug control laboratories and other competent institutions. This includes veterinary inspection and surveillance at the customer interface. It may not be an uncommon situation where a client describes a clinical problem in their animal, and after further questioning they reveal they have tried several human medicines or medicines purchased online prior to visiting the veterinarian. The diagnosis and treatment of animals lies solely with the veterinarian; for a non-veterinarian to undertake such a task is to potentially breach the Veterinary Surgeons Act 1966. Questioning clients at this stage may yield information as to where they obtained the medicine, and might also provide an opportunity for veterinarians to explain the risks of using medicines of unknown origins. Another potential route to curb the client's use of illegitimate medicine sources might be to introduce new entrepreneurial pricing practices and develop newer cost-effective treatments, eventually making the illegal trade no longer viable.

Conclusions

This chapter makes a contribution to both the veterinary practice and entrepreneurship literature by researching and documenting entrepreneurial behaviours and practices at the margins of the literatures on entrepreneurship and crime. Moreover, it documents another unusual application by setting entrepreneurship in a criminal context. In particular, the parallels between how the stereotypical images of veterinarians and entrepreneurs are socially constructed as heroes is a noteworthy angle. There is a need to challenge the old stereotypes and to formulate new stereotypes based on new roles and entrepreneurial ideology. There is also a pressing need for veterinarians, both individually and collectively, to embrace the ideology of entrepreneurship and to adopt a more entrepreneurial approach to restructuring their businesses and practices before industry outsiders and, more alarmingly, organized criminals take over the black market opportunities. Henry and Treanor (2010) argue that there is value in incorporating entrepreneurship education within the veterinary curricula to enhance students'

---

[16] Under the cascade in the VMR it is permissible for veterinarians to use unauthorized drugs too. This is very common due to the lack of VMs compared to the human equivalent.

employable skills and deliver on veterinary medicine's competences agenda. There is also value in educating and training veterinarians in how to spot and deal with examples of criminal entrepreneurship such as those focused upon in this chapter.

Summary

This chapter has introduced the possibility that the veterinary industry can become prey to unscrupulous and organized criminal entrepreneurs, and that there is a need to consider entrepreneurship in its many forms and to adapt to change in the industry. It has highlighted the need to examine practices and processes and to consider how to recognize and deal with examples of criminal entrepreneurship within the industry.

Review questions

1. Do you consider the veterinary practice in which you work or aspire to work to be an entrepreneurial practice?
2. Could it deal successfully with the issues discussed in this case?
3. Can you decipher the differences between legitimate and criminal entrepreneurship in an industry context?
4. Can you identify the links between entrepreneurship and criminal activity?
5. How would you arrange your practice to prevent your clients being enticed, even unknowingly, into illegitimate or criminal veterinary enterprises?

References

Alsos, G., Carter, S., Ljunggren, E., Welter, F. (Eds.), 2011. The Handbook of Entrepreneurship Research in Agricultural and Rural Development. Edward Elgar, Cheltenham, UK.

Arlacchi, P., 1986. Mafia Business: The Mafia Ethic and the Spirit of Capitalism. Verso, London.

Bailey, K., 1994. Documentary Research. Routledge, London.

Barclay, E.M., Donnermeyer, J.F., Jobes, P.C., 2004. The dark side of gemeinschaft: criminality within rural communities. Crime Prevention and Community Safety 6 (3), 7–22.

Barfield, C.E., Groombridge, M.A., 1999. Parallel trade in the pharmaceutical industry: implications for innovation, consumer welfare, and health policy. Fordham Intellectual Property Media and Entertainment Law Journal 185.

Baumol, W.J., 1990. Productive, unproductive, and destructive. Journal of Political Economy 98 (5): Part 1.

Brockhaus, R.H., 1980. Risk taking propensity in entrepreneurs. Acad. Manage. J. 23 (3), 509–520.

Brown, J., 2009. Veterinary forensics giving a voice to those who cannot speak for themselves. Honours thesis. Washington State University (accessed 16.01.13). Available: http://hdl.handle.net/2376/2422

Budge, A., Irvine, W., Smith, R., 2008. Crisis plan – what crisis plan? How rural entrepreneurs survive in a crisis. Journal of Small Business and Entrepreneurship 6 (3), 337–354.

Cooper, J.E., Cooper, M.E., 2008. Forensic veterinary medicine: a rapidly evolving discipline. Forensic Science, Medicine, Pathology 4 (2), 75–82.

Daughton, C.G., Ternes, T.A., 1999. Pharmaceuticals and personal care products in the environment: agents of subtle change? Environ. Health Perspect 107 (6), 907–938.

Davis, R.S., Potter, G.W., 1991. Bootlegging and rural criminal entrepreneurship. Journal of Crime and Justice 14 (1), 145–159.

Dean, S., 2009. Sales of medicines over the Internet. Vet. Rec. 164, 248–249.

De Silva, L.R., Kodithuwakku, S.S., 2011. Pluriactivity, entrepreneurship and socio-economic success of rural households. In: Alsos, G., Carter, S., Ljunggren, E., Welter, F. (Eds.), The Handbook of Entrepreneurship Research in Agricultural and Rural Development. Edward Elgar, Cheltenham, pp. 38–53.

Dingwall, G., Moody, S.R., 1999. Crime and Conflict in the Countryside. University of Wales Press, Cardiff.

Fitzgerald, T., 2007. Documents and documentary analysis: reading between the lines. In: Coleman, A.,

Briggs, A.R.J. (Eds.), Research Methods in Educational Leadership and Management. Sage, London, pp. 278–294.

Gauthier, D.K., 2001. Professional lapses: occupational deviance and neutralization techniques in veterinary medical practice. Deviant Behavior 22 (6), 467–490.

Gottschalk, P., 2009. Entrepreneurship and Organised Crime: Entrepreneurs in Illegal Business. Edward Elgar, Cheltenham, UK.

Gottschalk, P., Smith, R., 2011. Criminal entrepreneurship, white-collar criminality, and neutralization theory. Journal of Enterprising Peoples, Communities and Places in the Global Economy 5 (4), 300–308.

Grant, W., Greaves, J., 2009. State veterinarians: the construction of rural expertise in England. Paper prepared for the European Society for Rural Sociology Congress, Vaasa, Finland, 17–20 August 2009.

Green, S.P., 2006. Lying, Cheating, and Stealing: A Moral Theory of White Collar Crime. Oxford University Press, Oxford.

Hack, S., 2011. Enforcement of medicines regulations. Vet. Rec. 69, 589–590.

Hannah, H.W., 2002. The ethical content of veterinary medical practice acts. J. Am. Vet. Med. Assoc. 220 (5), 610–611.

PART ONE   Theoretical foundations
Henry, C., Treanor, L., 2010. Entrepreneurship education and veterinary medicine: enhancing employable skills. Education + Training 52 (8/9), 607–623.

Henry, C., Treanor, L., 2012. The veterinary business landscape: contemporary issues and emerging trends. In: Perez-Marin, C.C. (Ed.), Veterinary Medicine: A Bird's Eye View. InTech Publishing, New York, pp. 3–16 (accessed 16.01.13). Available: http://www.intechopen.com/books/a-bird-s-eye-view-of-veterinary-medicine/the-veterinary-business-landscape-contemporary-issues-and-emerging-trends

Henry, C., Baillie, S., Treanor, L., 2010. Encouraging women's entrepreneurship in the sciences: women in veterinary medicine. In: Wynarczyk, P., Marlow, S. (Eds.), Innovating Women: Contributions to Technological Advancement. Contemporary Issues in Entrepreneurship Research, Vol. 1. Emerald Group, Bingley, UK, pp. 15–33.

Henry, C., Baillie, S., Rushton, J., 2011. Exploring the future sustainability of farm animal veterinary practice. Paper presented at the 9th Rural Entrepreneurship Conference at Nottingham Trent University, June 2011.

Hobbs, D., 1988. Doing the Business: Entrepreneurship, the Working Class, and Detectives in the East End of London. Oxford University Press, Oxford.

Hoffman, B., Goericke-Pesch, S., Schuler, G., 2011. Antiprogestins, high potential compounds for use in veterinary research and therapy: a review. Eurasian Journal of Veterinary Sciences 27 (2), 77–96.

Iaquinto, A., Spinelli Jr., S., 2006. Never Bet the Farm: How Entrepreneurs Take Risks, Make Decisions – and How You Can, Too! Jossey-Bass, San Francisco, CA.

Kanavos, P., Costa-Font, J., 2005. Pharmaceutical parallel trade in Europe: stakeholder and competition effects. Economic Policy 20 (44), 751–798.

Kogan, L.R., McConnell, S.L., 2001. Gaining acceptance into veterinary school: a review of medical and veterinary admissions policies and practices. J. Vet. Med. Educ. 28 (3), 101–110.

Liang, B.A., 2005. Parallel trade in pharmaceuticals: injecting the counterfeit element into the public health. NC Journal of International Law and Commercial Regulation 31 (4), 847–900.

McElwee, G., 2006. Farmers as entrepreneurs: developing competitive skills. Journal of Development Entrepreneurship 11 (3), 187–206.

Malecki, E.J., 2006. Remarks at the Conference on Exploring Rural Entrepreneurship: Imperatives and Opportunities for Research. Washington, DC, 26–27 October 2006.

Mingay, G.E., 1989. The Rural Idyll. Routledge, London.

Mogalakwe, M., 2006. The use of documentary research methods in social research. African Sociological Review 10 (1), 221–230.

Nerlich, B., Hamilton, C.A., Rowe, V., 2002. Conceptualising foot and mouth disease: the socio-cultural role of metaphors, frames and narratives (accessed 25.02.08). http://www.metaphorik.de/02/nerlich.pdf

Platt, J., 1981. Evidence and proof in documentary research. Sociol. Rev. 29 (1), 31–52.

RCVS, 2012. Code of Professional Conduct for Veterinary Surgeons. Royal College of Veterinary Surgeons, London.

Sarasvathy, S.D., 2001. Causation and effectuation: towards a theoretical shift from economic inevitability to entrepreneurial contingency. Acad. Manage. Rev. 26 (2), 243–263.

Saugeres, L., 2002. Of tractors and men: masculinity, technology and power in a French farming community. Sociologia Ruralis 42 (2), 143–159.

Scott, J., 1990. A Matter of Record: Documentary Sources in Social Research. Polity Press, Cambridge, UK.

Scott, J., 2006. Documentary Research. Sage, London.

Sharma, M.C., Tiwari, R., Sharma, J.P., 2010. Entrepreneurship in Livestock and Agriculture. Vedams, New Delhi.

Smith, D.C., 1978. Organized crime and entrepreneurship. International Journal of Criminology and Penology 6 (2), 161–177.

Smith, R., 2004. Rural rogues: a case story on the smokies trade. International Journal of Entrepreneurial Behaviour and Research 10 (4), 277–294.

Smith, R., 2009. Understanding entrepreneurial behaviour in organised criminals. Journal of Enterprising Communities: People and Places 3 (3), 256–268.

Smith, R., 2010. Policing the changing landscape of rural crime: a case study from Scotland. International Journal of Police Science and Management 12 (3), 373–387.

Smith, R., McElwee, G., 2013. Confronting social constructions of rural criminality: a case story on 'illegal pluriactivity' in the farming community. Sociologica Ruralis 53 (1), 112–134.

Stearn, D.W., 2004. Deterring the importation of counterfeit pharmaceutical products. Food and Drug Legal Journal 59 (4), 537–561.

Sutherland, E.H., 1949. White Collar Crime. Dryden Press, New York.

Tannenbaum, J., 1995. Veterinary Ethics: Animal Welfare, Client Relations, Competition and Collegiality, second ed. Mosby, St Louis, MO.

Terzić, S., Šandor, K., Andrišić, M., et al., 2011. Counterfeit veterinary medicinal products: a potential threat. Veterinarianerinarska Stanica 42 (2), 175–180.

Windsor, R., 2002. What has happened to our institutions? Talk to the Central Veterinary Society.

Wright, J.G., 1961. The veterinary profession, past, present and future. 3: The future. Vet. Rec. 73 (10), 245–247.

Yin, R.K., 2003. Case Study Research: Design and Methods, third ed. Sage, London.

Documentary evidence

Author unattributed, 2011a. Veterinarian medicine market must be simpler. NFU, 16 June (accessed 10.01.13). Available: http://www.farmersguardian.com/home/livestock/livestock-news/veterinarian-medicine-market-must-be-simpler-nfu/39733.article

Author unattributed, 2011b. Lincolnshire pensioner admits part in £6 m drugs trade. Lincolnshire Echo,

9 July 2011 (accessed 10.01.13). Available: http://www. thisislincolnshire.co.uk/Lincolnshire-pensioner-admits-pound-6m-drugs/story-12913528-detail/story.html

Author unattributed, 2011c. Worcester pair sentenced over illegal animal medicines, 8 July 2011 (accessed 10.01.13). Available: http://www. birminghampost.net/news/west-midlands-news/2011/07/08/worcestershire-pair-sentenced-over-illegal-animal-medicines-65233-29020324/#ixzz1Wp3bX9tw

Author unattributed, 2011d. Guilty in £6 m veterinarian drugs scam. Evesham Journal 26 (5)(accessed 10.01.13) Available: http://www. eveshamjournal.co.uk/news/9047792.Guilty_in___6m_veterinarian_drugs_scam/

Author unattributed, 2011e. UK: veterinarians, drug companies and criminals, 13 July 2011 (accessed 10.01.13). Available: http://www. meattradenewsdaily.co.uk/news/130711/uk___veterinarians_drug_companies_and_criminals_.aspx

Author unattributed, 2011f. Country life couple jailed for Europe's biggest illegal veterinarian medicines scam, 10 July 2011 (accessed 10.01.13). Available: http://squaremilenews. blogspot.co.uk/2011/07/country-life-couple-jailed-for-europes.html

Author unattributed, 2011g. Worcestershire pair sentenced over illegal animal medicines. 8 July 2011 (accessed 10.01.13). Available: http://www.sundaymercury. net/news/midlands-news/2011/07/08/worcestershire-pair-sentenced-over-illegal-animal-medicines-65233-29

Author unattributed, 2011h. Farmer caught up in veterinary medicines scam is spared jail, 11 July 2011 (accessed 10.01.13). Available: http://www.meltontimes. co.uk/news/crime/farmer-caught-up-in-veterinarianerinary-medicines-scam-is-spared-jail-1-2854921

Boderke, D., 2012. Farmers warned over illegal veterinary medicines, 12 April, 2012 (accessed 10.01.13). Available: http://www.farmersguardian.com/home/latest-news/farmers-warned-over-illegal-veterinarianerinary-medicines/46188.article

Daily Mail Reporter, 2011a. Princess Diana lookalike's £13 m empire in illegal farm drugs. Daily Mail, 8 July 2011 (accessed 10.01.13). Available: article.wn.com/view/2011/07/08/Princess_Diana_lookalikes_13m_empire_in_illegal_farm_drugs/

Daily Mail Reporter, 2011b. Princess Diana lookalike and husband jailed for flooding UK (accessed 10.01.13). Available: http://article.wn.com/view/2011/07/07/Princess_Diana_lookalike_and_husband_jailed_for_flooding_UK_/

Driver, A., 2011. 13 convicted for £6 m veterinarian medicine smuggling, 13 July 2011 (accessed 10.01.13). Available: http://www. farmersguardian.com/home/livestock/livestock-news/13-convicted-for-%C2%A36m-veterinarian-medicine-smuggling/40167.article

nics.gov.uk, 2004. Trade in illegal veterinary products must stop – Smith, 22 December 2004 (accessed 10.01.13). Available: http://www.ergogenics.org/farmdrugs.html

Applying marketing theory to veterinary practice

7

Andrew Morton

CHAPTER OVERVIEW

As a specialized business discipline, marketing has grown in importance over the years. This chapter identifies and discusses some of the most important marketing concepts and frameworks that have been used to build long-term successful businesses and practices.

Considerable attention is paid in the chapter to the marketing planning process, with the key elements of a successful marketing plan discussed. The value of some of the more recent digital developments is explored, and consideration is given to how veterinary practice managers and owners may wish to incorporate these into their overall marketing mix. This includes specific digital marketing strategies and tools.

One of the most important elements of any marketing plan is measuring and monitoring its overall effectiveness. By continually measuring activity, the overall effectiveness of your marketing efforts can be improved over time. This chapter will discuss ways in which a practice may do this.

LEARNING OUTCOMES

After reading this chapter, students will be able to:
- Appreciate the importance of market segmentation analysis.
- Understand the value and measurement of setting suitable marketing objectives.
- Appreciate the roles of branding and digital marketing.
- Apply and adapt principal marketing concepts and frameworks for the benefit of a veterinary practice as part of an integrated marketing plan.

Introduction

While marketing is often misunderstood by business owners and managers, it remains one of the most powerful business disciplines. Unfortunately, for many vets, marketing is often seen as the process of organizing some 'advertising' or simply producing some 'leaflets' – processes that are often detached from the operational side of the organization. This may be a somewhat naïve view, and one that will surely limit the long-term success of the organization.

In most cases, successful veterinary practices appreciate the view that if they are to succeed in an ever-changing and increasingly competitive economic climate then they must start to consider their customers and what they are looking for. This might sound fairly straightforward, but in many instances the needs and wants of the customers are overlooked by internal issues and rivalries, all of which undermine the potential of the veterinary practice.

In its truest form marketing could be seen as the strategy and process of putting the customer at the heart of the organization and developing the business around their needs. The Chartered Institute of Marketing (www.cim.co.uk) defines marketing as

> The management process responsible for identifying, anticipating and satisfying customer requirements profitably.
>
> (Blood, 1976).

By dissecting this statement it becomes quite clear that 'marketing' should be more than simply a

© 2014, Elsevier Ltd.

functional role within an organization. Essentially, it is the responsibility of the whole practice from top to bottom, and without that commitment and understanding the potential is severely weakened.

For any organization wishing to adopt a strong 'marketing orientation' the implications are substantial. This might, for example, include the range of services you offer, whether or not you offer an out-of-hours emergency service, or an online service, an in-house laboratory or even separate cat and dog wards. It may even extend to the recruitment of specialist staff and to other products and services such as Pet Plans and small-animal food products. It may seem obvious, but by adapting your business to suit your market you will make it more appealing to customers.

This chapter discusses the essentials of marketing planning, the setting of marketing objectives and the importance of understanding consumer buying behaviour. The value of branding along with the growth and opportunities of digital marketing, including social media, are also explored. This chapter will therefore provide a flavour of marketing strategy and tactics that can help build a long-term sustainable business.

Marketing for all

Whether you are a larger national organization, a small local practice or a new practice with a strong entrepreneurial spirit, there is always a need for well-thought-out marketing. Many small veterinary practices suffer from a lack of finance, so embarking on an expensive advertising campaign might be out of the question. Likewise, you might have serious resource limitations, so starting a time-consuming social media campaign might be too much of a burden for already busy staff, or you might be too busy caring for clients, dealing with suppliers or worrying about the more mundane issues of managing a team of people to take time out to develop an effective marketing campaign. However, by investing in a well-balanced and detailed marketing programme your chances of reaching your goals will be increased considerably. Irrespective of the size of your practice or your ambitions, the core principles of any effective marketing campaign alter little.

Marketing and sales

The marketing and sales functions are often confused and sometimes assumed to be one and the same. Both functions have similar objectives and work synergistically through interrelated techniques, although the timescales do differ. However, over the past century, marketing has evolved. Its focus has moved from the short-term, transactional level to the long-term, relationship level. These days, when it comes to 'satisfying customer requirements profitably' most marketers think over the long term and consider the 'life time value' (LTV) of a customer as one of the main measurement tools. Understanding and measuring the LTV of a customer is important, and we will be discussing how you might go about this later in the chapter. The reality is that building long-term relationships with the 'right sort' of customers will always be more effective than attracting customers who only buy once and never return. So, how do we ensure that our marketing activity is effective? It should start with the development and agreement on what you are trying to achieve. The business should have an over-arching business plan that might include a 'mission statement', financial analysis and targets, including relevant information on other management disciplines such as IT (information technology), HR (human resources) or operations. The important thing is that for your marketing to be successful it should be based on the mission and objectives of the business plan and relate to the plans for the other parts of the organization. A marketing plan that is developed in isolation is likely to fail.

What is your plan?

First and foremost, your plan needs to consider all the factors that might have an impact on its success. These may be things that your practice can control or influence (called internal factors) but might also include those factors that are beyond your control, such as changes to the law, the economic climate or the activities of your competitors (often referred to as external factors).

There are many marketing planning models and some are very similar to those used in other disciplines. One of the most common is PR Smith's SOSTAC® model:

S = Situation analysis (or 'Where are we?')
O = Objectives (or 'What do we want to achieve?')
S = Strategy (or 'How are we going to get there?')

T = Tactics (or 'What tools are we going to use?')

A = Actions (or 'When is it all taking place?')

C = Controls (or 'How are we going to manage it and find out how well we have done?')

A simplified example is shown in Table 7.1.

Utilizing models such as SOSTAC® helps focus the efforts of everyone in the practice, and often acts as a point for internal discussion and agreement.

Who is your audience?

Understanding as much as possible about your audience is vital. Some people will see an obvious need for your products and services, while others will not. If the latter is the case, make sure you do not waste time and money trying to convince them to change their minds. You have to be quite ruthless in establishing the characteristics of your primary target market. Sometimes this is quite obvious, but in many cases it requires further research.

Using quantitative data is important when establishing your target audience. It is too easy to be convinced that you have a large enough market even though this is often based on hearsay and anecdotes. Depending on your resources you could conduct your own market research using one of the free online services such as SurveyMonkey (www.surveymonkey.com), or simply ask your customers to complete a questionnaire while in the waiting room.

Established research organizations such as Mintel and Keynote regularly produce reports on the UK pet market but they may be chargeable. The Chartered Institute of Marketing has a library service, and reports can be accessed and small portions copied under licence (see Chartered Institute of Marketing, 2012a). Alternatively, there are lots of websites providing information on the veterinary market. So, whether you are targeting businesses such as racing stables or families with small animals it really does not matter. The important thing is to appreciate their characteristics and what they are looking for. To help with this, you might refer to four over-arching criteria: geographic, psychographic, behavioural and demographic. Table 7.2 highlights some of the elements of each of these criteria.

Table 7.1 An illustration of the use of the SOSTAC® model

Criteria	Description
S = Situation analysis	You have noticed that customer numbers are dropping year on year. Fewer people in your town have small pets and your costs have increased but you do not want to simply pass them on to the customers because a new competitor has opened up nearby. Your customers think you do a good job but are becoming more cost conscious and are prone to 'shop around'. By understanding the broader factors that impact on your practice your planning will be more effective.
O = Objectives	Internally you agree to target current customers with a view to '*In 12 months, increasing the number of customers who come more than once by 50%*'.
S = Strategy	Using the 7Ps model, you develop a plan to build relationships and offer new services that differentiate you from the competition and appeal to your potential and current customers.
T = Tactics	You need to create awareness and interest in your new Pet Plan, so you consider advertising but also need to make it easy for customers to buy. This might include advertising, running a sales offer, sponsoring the dog show at the annual fair, or providing leaflets in the waiting room. It might need training for front-line staff as well as information posted on your website. When it comes to promoting your products and services, remember to follow Lewis's AIDA model: Awareness, Interest, Desire, Action!
A = Actions	After considering all these marketing tools you develop a schedule of activity for the next 12 months. Each element is costed and its effectiveness measured.
C = Controls	To ensure that you meet your set objectives you implement specific management and measurement techniques. This might include adapting a person's job description, using Google Analytics or integrating your sales ledger with a marketing database.

Source: Smith PR (2011) *SOSTAC® Guide to writing the perfect plan*, www.prsmith.org.

Table 7.2 Market segmentation criteria

Market segment criteria	Variables
Geographic	Rural, urban, local, national, international, etc.
Behavioural	Occasional/heavy use, loyalty status, attitudes, benefit sought
Psychographics	Social class, lifestyle, personality
Demographics	Age, income, education, family life stage

If you are targeting other businesses rather than individual pet owners, you may already have an idea of what your primary audience might be, but again it is worth identifying common characteristics. For example, you could investigate their current turnover, or the number of staff, or the number and location of practices in the whole group. You might also consider the business's decision-making and buying process. Do they have a tight procurement policy and, if so, are you in a position to meet their requirements? They may also have seasonal buying patterns. If so, are you able to take advantage of these?

By defining your target audience in detail you can adapt your marketing activity to make it more appealing and attractive. In targeting your audience, you should also consider additional factors such as number of employees, turnover, location, decision-making and procurement processes. Such considerations will allow you to identify and quantify your key market segments, and from there you can build effective marketing plans.

Consumer buying behaviour

Over the years there has been a lot of research exploring the process that individuals go through when in the 'buying process'. While the scale varies considerably depending on whether it is a 'big-ticket' item such as agreeing terms on a new practice, or smaller everyday products such as worm, flea and parasite treatments, as consumers we all follow a process. For marketers, understanding this process, and adapting marketing and communications activity accordingly, can increase the number of new customers as well as improving customer retention and loyalty. Figure 7.1 illustrates this process and identifies some key marketing tactics that need to be considered.

Often marketing campaigns focus on one or two aspects of the buying process, so it might be worth considering what strategies and tactics are available to you to ensure that you do not lose potential customers along the way. Most organizations are limited in their marketing communications activity at some stage through a lack of resources such as finance, skills, staff and time. It is worth analysing your available resources before making any serious commitments.

Positioning your products and services

For your marketing activity to really succeed you need not only to appreciate what your target market looks like, but also how you are viewed by that audience compared to your competitors. While you might think that what you are offering is unique, your target audience might simply see your company/ veterinary practice as just the same as any other. In this case it is vital to develop your competitive advantage and demonstrate how and why you are different. This differentiation can be made for all sorts of reasons but it must be appealing and relevant. There is no point in offering a 24/7 emergency service if your target market is not the least bit interested. Furthermore, your potential customers may tell you that 'low price' is important and that your competitors are cheaper than you. This may be true, but be wary; it may be that 'value for money' is what really counts to them, so check before entering a potential price war. Thus, how you differentiate yourself from the competition needs careful consideration. Whatever your choice, it has to be appealing and sustainable. It may also have implications for the whole practice, not just for the promotional messages you put out.

In his book, *Competitive Strategy: Techniques for Analysing Industries and Competitors*, Harvard University's Michael Porter (2004) suggests that an organization has three options with regard to marketing strategy: cost leadership, product differentiation and focus (on specific target audiences). Unfortunately many organizations, and small businesses/practices in particular, lack clear direction and tend to fall into 'no man's land', resulting in a weak and sometimes confusing *competitive advantage*. While there is a certain amount of flexibility in these options, having a clear and long-term view of the adopted strategy will help define the actual marketing activities you eventually select.

Figure 7.1 • The consumer buying process

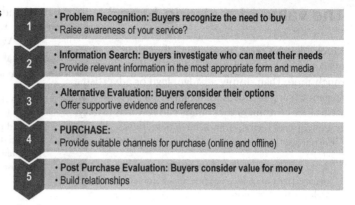

1
- **Problem Recognition: Buyers recognize the need to buy**
- Raise awareness of your service?

2
- **Information Search: Buyers investigate who can meet their needs**
- Provide relevant information in the most appropriate form and media

3
- **Alternative Evaluation: Buyers consider their options**
- Offer supportive evidence and references

4
- **PURCHASE:**
- Provide suitable channels for purchase (online and offline)

5
- **Post Purchase Evaluation: Buyers consider value for money**
- Build relationships

Defining your competitive advantage

Marketers suggest that to be successful you need to decode what your competitive advantage is and select your 'unique selling proposition' (USP) in the belief that having one advantage is better than having lots. However, as customers become more selective and markets become more fragmented, it is often wiser to develop more than one USP relevant to the different segments and micro markets. Unfortunately, taking this approach can sometimes lead to confusion. For example, if you identify five key points of difference, the issue then becomes: which one do you promote? Developing new promotional campaigns can be beneficial but can also be costly. So it may be worth researching which point resonates most with your target audience.

Your USP does not have to be related to specific features; it could relate to how you promote yourself/your practice, the levels of service and support you provide and the way you communicate with your customers and stakeholders. Whatever you decide, it must be appealing to your target customers; it is they who will decide whether or not it is of real interest.

Setting objectives

Taking into account the overall direction and business objectives should allow you to develop suitable marketing objectives. In many cases, business people view marketing as a 'cost' rather than a positive 'investment', and often need to be convinced of the possible benefits. By setting clear and measurable

objectives beforehand you are more likely to gain commitment from across the practice as well as approval for the activity.

What do you want to achieve?

Many objectives can be poorly devised, along the lines of being the 'biggest' or the 'need to sell more'. While these may demonstrate some underlying desire they are vague and somewhat difficult to measure. Therefore, when devising marketing objectives it is worth considering the SMART acronym. 'S' stands for 'specific', 'M' stands for 'measurable', 'A' stands for 'achievable', 'R' for realistic – do you have the resources and skills? The final 'T' stands for 'time-bound'. A useful example of a SMART objective might therefore be: *For the period March 2013 to February 2014 we will increase total sales value by 25%.* This example is quite simplistic and you might eventually have many objectives, each of which must be measurable. Units of measurement might be straightforward, such as pounds earned (return on investment or ROI) but could be far more complex. Customer services, public relations and social media in particular are quite difficult to measure as they might relate to factors such as 'reputation', 'usability' and 'buzz'.

With regard to your digital marketing, Dave Chaffey and P. R. Smith in their book *eMarketing eXellence* (2009) suggest using the 5 s model to develop the key online strategies and tactics, which include *Sell* (increasing sales), *Serve* (adding value), *Speak* (getting closer to customers), *Save* (reducing your costs), *Sizzle* (extending your brand online). In essence, all your digital activity should be trying to achieve one or all of these.

The value of a strong brand

Much like the term 'marketing', 'branding' is often overused and misunderstood. Essentially, a brand is much more than simply a badge, logo or advertising slogan. Strong brands have an emotional connection with their customers that builds and rewards loyalty. In conceptual terms, brands have been defined by de Chernatony *et al.* as

> A cluster of functional and emotional values that enables organisations to make a promise about a unique and welcomed experience.
>
> de Chernatony *et al.* (2011, p. 31)

However, the development of a successful brand takes time. Not only does it require the development of effective and appealing products and services, but also the manner in which they are promoted and supported. If you think of the world's biggest brands – Coca Cola, Apple, McDonalds, etc. – they are each well defined. Irrespective of whether or not you like the brand or understand the product specifications, you probably have an idea of what they do and what makes them different. Part of that difference will be emotional factors rather than defined products and product features. It is this combination of emotional and factual differences that defines the brand.

Most famous brands took time and considerable investment before they could be called 'established'. But more important than investment is the development of clear brand values that are easily recognizable and agreed by all your stakeholders such as staff, customers, suppliers, associates and the media. If, for example, you were to take one of your own favourite brands and dissect what makes it differ from its competitors it might give you an idea of what you should do for your own. The size of the advertising budget is certainly important, but what makes, for example, the Apple iPhone stand out against other mobile phone manufacturers? When you delve into it, the emotional factors (such as status, fashion and image) that drive people to buy the iPhone outweigh the technical ones. Establishing that emotional bond is vital in building strong brands.

Marketing strategies

The online revolution has had a tremendous effect on businesses of all sizes and from all sectors. It has resulted in consumers having more choice than ever before and, with the advent of social media, the freedom to interact with suppliers quickly and cheaply. While this has benefited many, it has also meant that the consumer can now complain openly about you and your products. As Scott claims:

> Prior to the Web: organizations had only two significant choices to attract attention: Buy expensive advertising or get third party ink from the media. But the web has changed the rules. The Web is not TV. Organizations that understand the New Rules of Marketing and PR develop relationships directly with consumers like you and me.
>
> Scott (2007, p. 5)

For marketers this means knowing more about media choices and understanding how and what media your customers use. These days, we all expect organizations to have websites and, in most cases, we expect to be able to buy online. However, consumers are now disappointed by simple static web pages, expecting some kind of interactivity such as video, free advice and access across all sorts of platforms including the social networks such as Facebook, Twitter and YouTube. Furthermore, they are accessing media on the move, searching and buying while on their mobiles, so sites have to be mobile friendly. Thus, whatever your product, your marketing plan must consider the online media options. No longer is online simply another route to market; no longer does online mean websites, email and SMS. Today it is mainstream, offering an online alternative to each traditional promotional activity. Whether it is simple brand and product advertising, sales promotions, direct marketing or public relations, online opportunities exist and are often very cost effective. If you are in any doubt about the value of digital marketing consider some of these benefits.

1. *Reach*: digital marketing allows you to reach new potential customers not constrained by time or location, and this can be done 24 hours a day, 365 days a year.
2. *Cost effective*: there are many digital tools and techniques that are either free or relatively cheap to use in your communications. Most offer a considerable degree of flexibility and level of customization. This efficiency also allows you to test different marketing concepts and messages to establish what works best.
3. *Immediacy*: unlike traditional media, digital marketing does not necessarily require weeks of preparation. For example, advertising on Google can be set by the hour, and the text can be changed within a few minutes.

4. *Personalization*: depending on the quality of the customer information you hold, you can develop any number of unique campaigns, each with different and highly targeted messages. This may require an initial investment in a suitable customer database but it will pay dividends in the end.

Strategy: the marketing mix

As we have seen, marketing is much more than a 'T-shirts and posters' function, and should have an impact across the whole organization from motivating and informing staff and stakeholders to generating new and profitable custom. For many leading marketers the cornerstone is the development of an appropriate marketing mix plan that incorporates seven aspects of the business. These are called the 7Ps – Product, Place, Price, Promotion, People, Processes and Physical Evidence – and require specific but integrated plans. Blythe (2008) defines the marketing mix elements as those depicted in Table 7.3.

The mix elements are interrelated, and changing one will have an impact on others. In some cases they might actually be seen as the responsibility of other departments such as finance or logistics, which may complicate and limit the effectiveness of the marketing activity. For many practices it is the Promotional 'P' that is most associated with marketing and marketing communications. It is this mix element upon which the remainder of this chapter will focus.

The promotional mix

Sometimes referred to as the 'marketing communications mix', this has become far more complex in recent years and, as we will see later, the advent of social media and smartphones has meant an explosion of promotional tools and options. Marketers across the country have to get to grips with new channels very quickly. However, even with this growth it is still considered that there are five major elements of the promotional mix, and it is worth considering the potential value of these for your veterinary practice (Table 7.4).

Deciding which tools to use and when is never easy and, for each traditional offline option, we now have to consider the online version as well. Getting your mix wrong can be an expensive exercise, so it is worth taking your time to get it right. If budget and time allow, it is also worth testing concepts, messages and media.

Arguably, one of the most effective promotional tools open to veterinary practices is the use of client

Table 7.3 The extended marketing mix

Mix element	Description
Product	The bundle of benefits the practice offers to customers. The element intended to meet people's needs. Could include both services and physical products.
Price	Goes beyond the cost to customers and includes all extras such as switching costs and training expenses.
Place	This is where the exchange takes place – practices, by mail, Internet etc. – and includes aspects of distribution and consumer convenience.
Promotion	This incorporates all the different promotional tools that might be used, including internal and external tactics.
People	Your front-line staff, delivering the services and handling complaints and queries. Often extending to other departments such as the laboratory, accounts and suppliers.
Physical evidence	The tangible aspects of the business; the practice decor, windows and vehicles. Each has an impact on customer perception.
Process	The systems affecting the relationship with customers, such as purchasing online, complaints procedures and client accounting.

testimonials. They are easy to generate and cost little to produce. For customers, particularly new customers, they offer a gentle reminder of your professional qualities and help overcome any concerns. However, you must take care and follow the proper procedure whenever canvassing for such material. The person providing the testimonial must be made fully aware of how you intend to use their testimonial and must agree to the actual wording used (see Chartered Institute of Marketing, 2012b, for further information).

Digital developments

In 1998, the marketing environment changed forever with the launch of a search engine called 'Google'. Since then brands like YouTube, Facebook and Twitter have significantly changed business processes.

Table 7.4 Key promotional tools

Promotional mix tools	Description	Key benefits
Advertising	Includes broadcast (TV, radio etc.), print, outdoor	Create awareness and interest. Reach wide audience
Direct marketing	Includes email, direct mail, SMS	Convey detail to specific individuals
Sales promotions	Includes in-store and online discounts, offers	Encourage purchase, overcome competition
Public relations	Includes corporate communications, press releases, events	Build brand credibility and reputation
Direct sales	Includes sales teams, online sales	Build relationships with decision makers

Today it is estimated that one in ten household pets have at least one picture on Facebook (www.telegraph.co.uk, 2012), and even the ubiquitous *Farmers Weekly* now includes blogs and forums on their website (www.fwi.co.uk). The Royal College of Veterinary Surgeons is also on Twitter (@rcvs_uk) and offers email updates through its RSS feeds.

As individuals and as businesses we have not only started 'searching' but we are now 'following', 'tweeting' and 'linking' with all sorts of people. The effect has been so dramatic that we have even invented a new language. Today we are worrying about brand 'buzz', 'sentiment' and 'passion'. Some special consumers have even now become 'prosumers'!

Essentially, organizations are slowly coming to realize that there has been a shift in the relationship between company and consumer; control is moving away from the company to the consumer. Customers are now the ones telling organizations what products and services to provide, how they want to receive information and how they prefer to pay. However, there is a very substantial benefit here; if managed correctly, these customers will ultimately become your brand advocates, championing your cause to all their friends and colleagues. We have referred to 'word of mouth' for years, but its importance is much greater in the digital age.

In effect, the way we think about marketing has changed completely in the last ten years, and the expectation is that this change will continue into the future. The introduction and convergence of new technologies such as smartphones, cloud computing and improved online security have led to a vast range of new products and channels for business. Moreover, these new technologies are often free to use, adopting 'freemium' pricing structures, where the basic version is free and charges are made for more complex versions. The result is that even the smallest of businesses can utilize digital tools without incurring excessive costs. For example, by keeping a record of your customer email addresses and mobile phone numbers you could quite easily arrange for them to receive messages and texts when it is time for their pets to receive their vaccinations and boosters. Furthermore, the traditional marketing planning process highlighted above is still very relevant and possibly even more significant in the long term. However, in the short term there are two key digital developments that are likely to have a greater impact than any other – mobile and social media – so it is worth discussing them individually.

The role of mobile marketing

For many people, the days of a mobile phone being simply a device to make a call while out of the house or office have been consigned to history. Mobile (including tablet) technology incorporates so much more, from high-quality touch screens to inbuilt GPS and WiFi, to voice recognition and video. The mobile phone is no longer a single-function device and consumers have been quick to realize this. Recent research (Mashable.com, 2011) in the USA suggests, for example, that around 40% of smartphone and tablet owners use their devices while watching TV. The research suggests that more than half were checking emails while around 40% were surfing the web or visiting social network sites.

The smartphone in particular has led to multitasking not only while watching TV but in the workplace, the supermarket or away on business. The smartphone is often the first place we go to when we are looking for information, advice or to buy. Consumers are no longer satisfied if they cannot get the information they want on their mobiles. Businesses have so many options these days it is sometimes hard to decide on the correct action to take. However, as a starting point, having a mobile-ready website is probably a wise decision. Google suggest that around 60% of mobile users are unlikely to return to a website that they have had trouble accessing. Furthermore, they also suggest that 41% will go to one of your competitors instead. For anyone concerned about attracting and retaining customers this must be of great concern. Fortunately, the cost of setting up a mobile-friendly website is not excessive. Google (2011) themselves offer a simple mobile template to get you going (for more information see http://www.google.com/sites/help/mobile-landing-pages/mlpb.html). Additionally, you might also consider the value of developing an 'app' or software application. Often considered as a product for the entertainment or online gaming sector, apps are proving very important in the commercial sector as well. Depending on your overall marketing objectives and strategy, an app might play a valuable role in building and maintaining relationships with your target market while enhancing your reputation.

Social media: 'flash in the pan' or strategically important?

With almost one billion users and a market valuation of $50 billion, it is fair to say that Faceboook is unlikely to disappear in a hurry. While networks such as MySpace and Bebo have struggled in the past, networks such as Twitter, Linkedin and Facebook are well established in the daily lives of many of us. Indeed, Erik Qualman (2012), acclaimed author of *Socialnomics*, went as far as saying: 'We do not have a choice on whether we do Social Media, the question is "how well do we do it?"' The implication is quite simple; if you want your business to be around in five years you need to join the social media community and quickly (see also Qualman's YouTube video: http://www.youtube.com/watch?v=x0Enh Xn5boM).

For many, the likes of Facebook and Twitter are a step too far, especially for a veterinary practice. They are far from being 'free', requiring considerable time and resources to manage properly and, without a proper strategy and appropriate internal business structures, can end up being more of hindrance than a valuable tool. One of the biggest issues relates to the perceived value of a presence on a social network. Will it bring in sales or simply give disgruntled customers yet another avenue to complain? For some time the jury has been out on how you can measure the effectiveness of your social media activity in comparison with more traditional forms of marketing communications such as direct mail or TV and radio advertising. However, this is changing with the realization that one of the main drivers for social media is building and maintaining strong brand 'values', 'reputation' and in some cases 'personality'. Unfortunately, these can be quite difficult to measure, especially in the context of social networks, but there are new services being launched almost daily and the networks themselves provide useful support. Ultimately, though, social media will have an impact on your practice, so make sure that you adhere to the now established protocols: listen to people first, provide advice and information for free, be polite and react to complaints and issues quickly, be honest and open and, possibly the most important, do not try to sell, ever! Setting up a company Facebook page, for example, would allow you to engage with customers about all sorts of things such as changes to opening hours; answer questions and provide advice; post 'lost and found pets' notices and invite customers to add their favourite pets' photos. They may appear to be only small things but collectively they help build a rapport with your customers.

Integrated marketing communication

It often happens – the Friday afternoon telephone call or email from a newspaper or radio station offering you an unbelievable deal on the next edition or slot: massive coverage at a knock-down price. In some cases the deal on offer might be worth it, but the reality is that unless the opportunity can be justified against your primary target audience and key objectives it is probably a 'punt to nothing'. For the majority, long-term sustainability is vital, and advertising should play an important role in attracting new customers and reminding current customers of the benefits of dealing with you. However, it cannot happen overnight.

Two critical factors should be considered when buying advertising. Firstly, will the media 'reach' the right type of people who might be interested in your services? Secondly, and perhaps more importantly, will the advertising campaign be repeated enough times for the message to actually be seen/heard amongst all the other advertising messages, and, perhaps more importantly still, will the key messages be understood? Exactly how many times must an advert appear before the right people actually see and read it is debatable, but a best guess might be between three and eight times. So the chance of anybody in your target audience seeing a 'one-off' advert, taking in the message and acting on it is not great, and probably not worth the effort.

These two aspects – 'reach' and 'frequency' – are fundamental to the success of any marketing communications campaign. Fortunately, your campaign does not need to rely solely on expensive TV, radio and print advertising. By researching your media options and using these channels selectively in an integrated manner you will be more effective and reduce wastage. There are many media tools to help you, such as ALF Business Development and BRAD Media Planning (www.bradinsight.com). Additionally, when it comes to online campaigns you could consider Google and Yahoo. Both provide a huge amount of material relating to the internet and campaigns.

By using a combination of tools in a coordinated and structured manner even the smallest business can find success. In many cases this can be done by using relatively inexpensive tools such as Internet and email, public relations and events. However, before you commit to one form of communications, it is probably wise to test not only the medium but the message as well. Table 7.5 shows examples of relatively cost-effective media open to all.

For all promotional activity there is a cost in terms of time and/or money. Some things you will be able to do regularly and others not. It is therefore important to develop a schedule of activity. At the very least it will provide a focus for the practice, taking into account relevant issues such as production times, staff resources and local market conditions. Table 7.6 shows a typical six-month schedule.

Developing the right message

Having the most detailed media plan is only half the story. These days it is important that you have a creative concept which is appealing to your target audience. Unfortunately, the introduction of desktop publishing and in-house design and production has resulted in a greater number of campaigns, but many of these are based on poor creative concepts. Good creativity is something worth paying for. Whether it is a compelling press release, an enticing website or an inspiring advert, developing the creative content is often best left to the professionals.

When it comes to creativity one useful framework is the DRIP acronym, which stands for *Differentiate, Remind, Inform* and *Persuade*. Essentially, DRIP suggests that whatever actions you decide upon they should all work together to make your practice stand out, attracting new clients and retaining existing ones. While creating awareness and generating a strong brand reputation is usually a critical objective, one of the most overlooked aspects of marketing communications is the 'call to action'. In essence you should try to make it as easy as possible for potential customers to contact you via their preferred communication choice. For example, this may include a website and email address, a Facebook or Twitter link, or a simple phone number.

Table 7.5 Examples of online promotional tools

Communications	Tool	Sources
Advertising	Pay per click (you only pay for the clicks through to your website or bespoke landing page)	Google Adwords Yahoo
Public relations	News releases: online and printed versions Journalist visits/open days Events and conferences Online 'content marketing' for social networks Corporate and personal blogs Forums and online discussions	National, regional and local media Facebook, Twitter, Youtube, Flickr, LinkedIn, etc.
Direct marketing	Email and online newsletters, direct mail	
Sales promotions	Introductory offers, discounts, off-peak incentives	
Face-to-face selling	Online virtual assistant, call centre	

Table 7.6 Tactical marketing schedule

Activity	Notes	Jan.	Feb.	Mar.	Apr.	May	June
Website	Ongoing	X	X	X	X	X	X
Virtual assistant	Ongoing	X	X	X	X	X	X
News release	Not during school holidays		X			X	
Blog updates/responses	Weekly	X	X	X	X	X	X
Email offers (dormant customers)	6 × per year	X		X		X	
E-newsletter	5 × per year to current/non-customers		X		X		X
Press day	Local and regional press			X			
Open day	Customers						X
Advertising	Trade magazines (3-insert deal)				X	X	X
Advertising	Local papers		X	X	X		
Events	County show × 2					X	X
Corporate literature	Leaflet flyers		X			X	

However, you need to bear in mind the changing behaviour of consumers – if, for example, your phone cannot be attended 24 hours a day, then link it to an answer-phone and try to respond the next day.

The development of a successful marketing campaign is complex, requiring strong planning and management skills, apart from excellent creativity. To assist you, some of the key points to remember are identified below:

1. Each tool and technique used should work to achieving the common objectives.
2. Remember that customers buy 'benefits and value', not 'features'. The benefits include emotional as well as practical ones.
3. Keep the messages simple and straightforward. It is too easy to over-complicate things by adding another feature and benefit.
4. Consider investing in high-quality creativity, copywriting and photography from professionals.
5. Be different and appealing!

Measuring success

As already indicated in this chapter, marketing should support the overall goals of your business. By establishing appropriate SMART objectives at the very start of any marketing activity you will be able to assess how effective your efforts have been. Perhaps more importantly, the measurement data and information will assist in the refining and enhancing of your marketing in the future. Marketing is a cyclical process, and whatever we learn should be used to improve our efforts in the future.

On the face of it, measuring might sound relatively easy. Integrated marketing campaigns can be quite complicated, with a number of different activities taking place, and identifying which of these is actually making a difference can be difficult. Similarly, understanding who actually purchased which of your services can be very useful information, helping you define your target audience and appreciate your customers' motivations. However, what may be even more important than your successes is finding out why people did not buy from you. It could be that your competitors made a better offer, the customer did not find the purchasing process easy or was unaware of your range of services. Whatever their reasons, it is vital that this information is gathered and analysed. There are many ways you can do this. You could consider using market research techniques such as quantitative and qualitative methods (e.g. customer surveys and interviews) or you might investigate your competition in a structured manner using set criteria so that you can establish rankings and points of differentiation. In this regard, data from the online world are readily available and in most cases are free (or very reasonably priced) to use. For example, Google Analytics (www.google.com/analytics/) will not only provide data on your website visitors but can also be linked to email campaigns. In the past, marketers were satisfied with just knowing visitor numbers, but these days we need to know much more. For example, by what route did the visitors come to the site and where did they go afterwards? How long were they on each page and which pages were the busiest? If you have an online shop it is also worth knowing how many people started buying but dropped out at some stage.

Fortunately, it is quite easy to test variations in terms of content and structure and to find the most effective options. So, even though the website is fully functioning, why not test a few options with regard to titles, images and content to see if you can improve?

Social media, on the other hand, are somewhat more difficult to measure, possibly because of the criteria used. Over the past few years, there has been much confusion over the value of social media. For many practices, the real value of social media may well have nothing to do with immediate and direct sales. Rather, it may be an important tool in building your brand reputation and personality, not unlike traditional PR. Websites such as Klout (www.klout.com) and Socialmention (www.socialmention.com) provide scores in relation to your level of 'influence', 'sentiment' and 'passion'. These scores reflect not only how much you are being discussed but also whether it is positive or negative. All this information is vital in improving consumer attitudes and affecting behaviour.

Delivering your marketing success

Embarking on an integrated marketing campaign such as that described above requires resources, and for small veterinary practices this might mean a trade-off with other work. However, having a marketing plan that has been agreed by everyone in the practice should help focus your efforts. Similarly, by establishing clear objectives the chances of getting distracted by less important activities will be reduced. How you manage your marketing activities is down to the individuals in the practice, but the following may be worth considering:

1. Allocating the marketing responsibility to a senior partner or director.
2. Using your marketing schedule to plan your workload.
3. Utilizing outside agency/consultancy support, especially at the start.
4. Using 'free' or cost-effective online services wherever possible, including email providers such as Mailchimp (www.mailchimp.com) and Constant Contact (www.constantcontact.com), who offer a range of email templates.
5. Building relationships with the media. (Press PR is still a very important tool in promoting businesses and it is relatively cheap.)
6. Testing your ideas before committing people and money. Remember, some ideas will work and others not.
7. Starting slowly and aiming to become more efficient over time; this is especially true for social media.

Conclusions

Marketing plays a vital role in building and maintaining a sustainable business, including a veterinary practice. Marketing strategies have an impact across all business functions, unlike any other management discipline. The advent of the Internet, digital marketing and social media means that traditional marketing practices are being challenged every day (Waldman, 2012). Nowadays, customers have much more choice and, through modern media such as Facebook and Twitter, a free public gallery to vent their anger if they feel let down. Ultimately, success means appreciating these changes, identifying your target customer groups and developing suitable programmes for each of those in a truly integrated fashion.

Summary

In the future, marketing will play an increasingly greater role for many veterinary practices. Increasing competition and changing consumer needs mean that practices should adapt. The marketing processes, concepts and frameworks discussed in this chapter provide an outline for practices to consider in their quest for improved efficiency and marketing effectiveness.

Review questions

1. In planning terms, what does SOSTAC® stand for?

2. The 'marketing mix' is widely regarded as the mainstay of a good marketing plan and is often referred to as the 7Ps. What are the 7Ps?

3. In the 'promotional mix', five promotional tools are identified. What are they?

4. Give one example of a relevant 'call to action' that you might use in a veterinary practice.

5. How might you measure the effectiveness of a social media campaign for a veterinary practice?

References

Blood, P., 1976. Chartered Institute of Marketing Annual Report. Chartered Institute of Marketing, Cookham, UK.

Blythe, J., 2008. Essentials of Marketing, fourth ed. Prentice Hall, Upper Saddle River, NJ.

Chaffey, D., Smith, P.R., 2009. eMarketing eXcellence. Butterworth-Heinemann, Oxford.

Chartered Institute of Marketing, 2012a (accessed 04.06.12.). Available: www.cim.co.uk/resources/productsandservices

Chartered Institute of Marketing, 2012b. Code of Professional Practice (accessed 05.11.12). Available: http://cim.co.uk/Files/codeofprofessionalstandards10.pdf

de Chernatony, L., McDonald, M., Wallace, E., 2011. Creating Powerful Brands. Butterworth-Heinemann, Oxford.

Google, 2011. Mobile-ize your site with Google Sites, Google Mobile Ads Google Blog. [4 June 2012].

Mashable.com, 2011. How people use smart phones and tablets while watching TV (accessed 04.06.12.). www.Mashable.com

Porter, M.E., 2004. Competitive Strategy: Techniques for Analyzing Industries and Competitors. Free Press, New York.

Scott, D.M., 2007. The New Rules of Marketing & PR. Wiley, Chichester, UK.

Smith, P.R., 2011. SOSTAC® guide to writing the perfect plan (accessed 10.01.13.). Available:www.prsmith.org

Qualman, E., 2012. Socialnomics: how social media transforms the way we live and do business. Wiley, Chichester, UK.

Waldman, S., 2012. Creative Disruption: What You Need to Do to Shake Up Your Business in a Digital World. Financial Times Series, Harlow, UK.

Brand identity: building a veterinary hospital brand

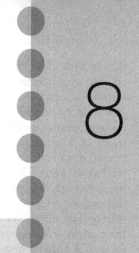

8

Catherine Coates

CHAPTER OVERVIEW

Brands and branding are marketing strategies, which were originally designed to promote the sale of physical goods through building customer loyalty. Over the past ten years, however, the branding approach has been adapted for application to service-based businesses. The use of branding to promote veterinary services is a relatively recent development, and the potential benefits that can be gained from the use of branding by veterinary practices and hospitals are not yet fully understood. This chapter draws on a range of published sources and research in other sectors to explain the brand concept, and discusses three key dimensions of branding: brand identity, brand values and brand equity. The application of these concepts to services, particularly to small and medium-sized service-based businesses (SMEs), is explored in order to gain insights into ways in which the strategy might be applied within the veterinary sector. Finally, the insights gained are brought together to put forward a theoretical model for rebranding a veterinary hospital.

LEARNING OUTCOMES

After reading this chapter, students will be able to:
- Explain the concepts of brand, brand identity, brand values and brand equity.
- Understand the differences between physical goods and services branding.
- Explain 'corporate branding' and why this approach is relevant to services.
- Outline an approach to branding a veterinary hospital.

Introduction

The use of brands and branding as a marketing strategy to promote veterinary services and build client loyalty is a relatively recent development in the UK. At the time of writing, published material on the subject is limited, and there is no veterinary-context-specific research on the effectiveness of branding or the extent to which it is applied within the industry. Although the concept has been embraced by corporate veterinary practices and others (e.g. Vets4Pets and Companion Care), it appears to be generally poorly understood in its implementation, which often extends merely to the use of symbols, such as logos, the choice of corporate colour schemes and/or external image and signage.

Branding is a complex, multifaceted marketing strategy, which was originally developed by large organizations as a means of uniquely differentiating physical goods, which were often very similar to each other. Originally, branding was not considered applicable to services or to small or medium-sized enterprises (SMEs: >50 and <250 employees, turnover not exceeding €50 million; EC SME Recommendation 2003/361/EC). Over time, however, as awareness of the power of brands and branding grew, the application of branding has become ubiquitous – extending outwards to embrace small organizations as well as service-based businesses.

The purpose of this chapter is to formulate an approach to building a veterinary hospital brand, which may be of use to owners and managers who wish to develop their own hospital's unique offering through

© 2014, Elsevier Ltd.

the use of branding. The first section, 'What is a brand?' explains what branding is and explores the meaning of three key concepts: 'brand identity', 'brand values' and 'brand equity'. 'Branding services' explains how branding principles are applied to services by drawing on the work of key researchers who have significantly advanced our understanding of services branding over the last ten years. The specific challenges involved in the use of branding within SMEs are then discussed, drawing out relevant lessons for veterinary managers who operate mostly within SMEs in the UK. Within the context of 'corporate branding', two examples of successful hospital brands within the UK and US health service sectors are discussed. These serve to demonstrate how effective branding can create powerful identities and can shape the entire culture and ethos of a hospital, leading to positive and lasting customer perceptions. Finally, an approach to branding a veterinary hospital is proposed, as an example of how corporate branding might be implemented within the veterinary services sector.

What is a brand?

Even though brands are ubiquitous, forming an integral part of most people's lives, there is no one commonly agreed definition of the concept. Definitions vary depending on the perspective from which the concept is viewed and the underlying philosophical stance taken (Wood, 2000). Thus a brand may be defined from the consumer's perspective, the brand owner's perspective or in terms of its purpose or characteristics, amongst others. For example, from the consumer's perspective, a brand may be defined as

> A set of instantly recognizable features and attributes, which bring the promise of quality, assurance, satisfaction and/or status.

From the brand owner's perspective, the definition might be

> Any one or a combination of symbol, name, design, catchphrase, word or sign intended to uniquely identify the product and differentiate it from similar competitor products.

Keller and Lehmann (2006) define brands from the point of view of their key functions and levels of impact. Thus the function of brands is to serve as markers or identifiers for a company's offerings, to simplify consumer choice, to reduce consumer risk and to build trust.

Brands are constructed starting with the core product, proceeding through the type and level of marketing activity undertaken to promote the product and, finally, to the consumer response to this marketing activity, as expressed by consumer purchasing behaviour. The impact of brands therefore occurs at three distinct levels: the core product or service, the consumer and the organization. The benefits accrued at each of these levels build the value of the brand, which is referred to as 'brand equity'. For example, with a can of Coca Cola®, benefits are accrued as follows:

- The product itself – is of good quality and consumers generally like the taste, which remains consistently pleasant and refreshing. Regular consumers of Coca Cola® can therefore rely on this quality and do not risk disappointment.
- The consumer – responds favourably to advertising, chooses this brand in preference to any other and is generally loyal to it.
- The organization – knows the consumer, matches the advertising and marketing campaigns with consumer preferences and needs and creates favourable impressions associated with the product (outdoor, sunshine, friendship, for everyone).

With successful brands, such as Coca Cola®, the benefits accrue not just to the organization that owns the brand but also to the consumer, and it is this mutual benefit that builds the value of the brand. Therefore, brands have also been described as 'intangible assets' that bring financial benefits to their owners and psychological rewards to consumers. Buying branded products is seen to bring additional benefits in the form of status, prestige or security, which unbranded products do not (Berthon *et al.*, 1999).

Pringle and Gordon (2001) provide a succinct definition of a brand as representing 'promises' about what one can expect from a product. According to the authors, brands combine both functional and rational attributes, as well as emotional and psychological imagery. The functional and rational attributes concern the product itself – the tangible features and functions that deliver value to the customer and which are unique. Emotions are evoked by the tone, style and imagery of the marketing communications promoting the product.

A number of associated concepts have emerged, which describe additional dimensions of branding and which serve to underline its complexity. Three key concepts are brand identity, brand values and brand equity.

Brand identity

Aaker (1996) defines brand identity as the combined effect of all of the external, visible features of a brand which are perceived by consumers, hopefully in the exact way that is intended by the organization which created it. In order to create brands, organizations first develop a 'vision' of what they want their brands to stand for and represent. In other words, they must create a brand's unique identity. Brand identity combines within it the organization's own values and beliefs, as well as the interests and needs of its customers. Brand identity is therefore an aggregation of what the organization represents and the expectations of its customers and is built upon an ongoing relationship with customers. Key aspects of brand identity, therefore, are the unique symbols, logos, phrases, tunes or trademarks that are used to represent the brand and which customers instantly recognize and associate with it. Examples of brands which have created their own unique identities are Nike, the Body Shop and McDonalds, where the products sold reflect company values and closely match the needs, lifestyles or aspirations of consumers.

Brand values

Successful brands are underpinned by a consistent set of brand values. These are the beliefs, aspirations and attitudes that describe and define the brand and differentiate it from others. Clearly identifiable brand values are an extension of the internal values of an organization, which enable the people working within it to understand how they should behave. This is particularly relevant to services, because by espousing the company's values employees are more likely to reflect these in their interactions with customers. If brand values are to be sustained, however, they must be delivered consistently, both internally and externally. For example, an organization that claims to value quality must ensure that this is delivered throughout its entire operation – in its premises, advertising, staff training and conduct, and in the quality of customer care (Jobber, 2001). The concept of brand values reflects the key principle that for a brand to be successful the values that it represents must be those of the organization itself and must underpin the functioning of that organization. Figure 8.1, which shows an adaptation of Davidson's (1997) 'branding iceberg', illustrates this principle. Davidson's original diagram has been adapted for the purposes of this chapter to show its relevance to services as well as products.

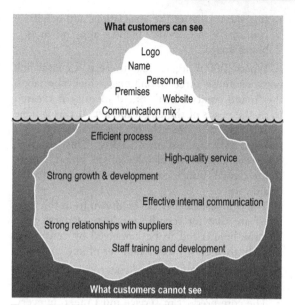

Figure 8.1 • The services branding 'iceberg'
Reproduced with permission from Davidson H. Even More Offensive Marketing, London, Penguin Books Ltd.; 1997.

According to Davidson (1997), what the customer sees and experiences is only the tip of the brand iceberg, which must be effectively underpinned by internal processes, communications and ways of working, which the customer does not see, but which must fully support the brand. Unsuccessful brands fail often because of internal inconsistencies, or because the promises that are made are not fulfilled. Berthon *et al.* (1999) argue that only strong and genuine brands will survive, because customers are now much more sophisticated and cannot be so easily persuaded. Customers have access through the Internet to considerably more information about brands than was previously available, enjoy greater purchasing power and are, consequently, much less loyal to brands than they used to be.

Brand equity

Feldwick (1996), as cited by Wood (2000), offers several different meanings for the concept of brand equity:

- Brand equity is the total value of a brand as an asset when it is sold or included in a company's balance sheet.
- It is a measure of the strength of consumers' attachment to a brand – also known as brand loyalty.

- It is the totality of the associations and beliefs consumers have about a brand – also known as brand image.

Wood (2000) argues that there is a causal link between these three definitions, which she labels the 'brand equity chain'. Brand identity is created to fit the needs of the target market. If this is done effectively, the strength of the brand increases through growing customer loyalty. This, in turn, determines the financial value of the brand, which, if substantial, brings competitive advantage to the brand owner.

The conclusions that can be drawn from the foregoing are that for specific products or services to become brands and to be perceived by consumers as such, they must meet a number of key criteria:

- They must be unique or distinctive and be recognized as such by consumers.
- The core product or service must meet, in every respect, the claims made about it by the supplier or service provider.
- Brands must bring significant additional benefits both to the consumer and the supplier/provider, which cannot be obtained from unbranded products or services.
- They must bring competitive advantage to the supplier/provider.
- They must be underpinned by a set of values, which are delivered consistently, both internally and externally, by the organization.
- They must consistently and actively build positive associations and foster consumer loyalty.

How can this level of differentiation and competitive advantage be achieved by providers of veterinary services? Veterinary services are generally considered by clients to be broadly of a similar type and quality, irrespective of marketing effort. While differentiation on the service alone might be difficult, it is possible to gain an advantage in a variety of other ways, focusing more on how the service is delivered.

Branding services

According to de Chernatony and Dall'Olmo Riley (1999), although most countries can now be defined as service economies, research on branding has hitherto been predominantly concerned with physical goods or products. De Chernatony and Dall'Olmo Riley (1999) considered whether the brand concept could also apply to services. Their research, involving interviews with brand experts, led to the conclusion that brands and branding are equally applicable to services, but that it is in the execution of the brand strategy where the differences between products and services become apparent because services branding requires a shift in marketing emphasis to take account of the specific characteristics of services.

Services are intangible in that they cannot be touched, seen or handled; rather, they are usually experienced. It is not possible to separate production and consumption of services, as it is with products. The quality of the service is entirely dependent on the people delivering it, on their knowledge, skills and abilities, and so the role of service personnel is crucial. De Chernatony and Dall'Olmo Riley (1999) reviewed the available literature and synthesized a number of proposed services branding strategies, as determined by services characteristics. These are summarized in Table 8.1.

Most of these strategies are primarily concerned with the effective promotion of the service brand and not with differentiating it from similar competitor offerings, which is a key function of brands. Consequently, if hospital managers were to adopt any one or several of these strategies, they may not necessarily gain competitive advantage. However, the corporate branding strategy, where the company or business itself is the brand, could potentially give the necessary competitive advantage because it is a holistic, relationship-based strategy. Dall'Olmo and de Chernatony (2000) support this view and put forward the concept of the service brand as a holistic construct, which focuses on the internal relationship between the company and its employees, which is enacted in the consumer–service-provider encounter.

Thus corporate branding encompasses all of the activities of a business, both internal and external. Key features of corporate branding include:

- Internal marketing – brand values and strategies are communicated to all staff so that they understand the company ethos and what it stands for.
- Training of front-line staff to ensure that they personify the brand to clients.
- Corporate identity which articulates the company's ethos, values and aims.
- Consistent communications to establish a favourable impression with clients and other stakeholders.

If a veterinary hospital could successfully achieve complete congruence between its own espoused

Table 8.1 Characteristics of services and suggested branding strategies

Service characteristic	Branding strategy
Intangibility	Build reputation through stimulating word-of-mouth recommendations Promote the company itself as the brand, i.e. corporate branding Use distinctive logos and/or physical facilities that can be clearly associated with the service provided Provide tangible cues that make the service more easily understood by clients
Inseparability	Select and train front-line staff to deliver the service brand Promote the company as the brand Build brand relationships by encouraging greater client participation in deciding the way the service is delivered
Heterogeneity	Customize the brand to serve the needs of specific clients better Apply 'internal branding', i.e. develop internal company values that support the service brand and that are delivered consistently Develop a 'service culture' Build good employee relations and effective internal communication systems
Perishability	Implement efficient systems and processes Deliver on promises about quality, speed and value for money Build company's image and reputation Reaffirm client's choice Maintain ongoing client relationships post purchase

Source: Adapted from de Chernatony and Dall'Olmo Riley (1999).

values, its employees' values and those of its clients, then it would create a strong corporate brand genuinely appreciated by clients.

In support of the corporate branding approach, De Chernatony and Segal-Horn (2001) argue that services branding strategies need to attend more to internal company issues than is the case with products, and specifically point to the importance of internal communications. They contend that while product branding focuses primarily on the consumer, successful services brands focus on all the stakeholders, especially the staff. Thus successful services companies employ people whose values concur with their own, so that they behave in a way that fulfils the 'brand promise'. A key finding of their research is that services brands are built upon a relationship between the brand and the consumer, which is developed through greater consumer dialogue and the integration of consumers into brand delivery processes. Furthermore, services brands are more likely to succeed if service delivery staff can build consumers' trust through genuine rather than superficial relationships.

Berry (2000) supports the corporate branding approach as most suitable for services branding, arguing that in the context of services, especially labour-intensive service businesses, the company is the primary brand, where human performance plays a critical role in building the brand. The intangibility of services and the key role of service personnel focus the customer's attention on the company as an entity, and so the company as a whole is viewed as the source of the customer's experience and hence becomes the locus of brand formation. Service companies build strong brands by

- performing their core service better than their competitors;
- reaching customers emotionally, capturing and communicating values that are dear to them;
- associating their brands with trust – providing truthful, honest and genuine experiences;
- consistent customer communications.

Two examples of successful corporate brands are Great Ormond Street Hospital (GOSH) in London, UK, and the Mayo Clinic in the USA.

GOSH (www.gosh.nhs.uk) relies on public donations. It has developed a reputation for excellence in clinical care and is the leading children's hospital in the UK. GOSH's fundamental values are encapsulated in its motto: *'The child first and always'*. It has clearly stated priorities of *'safety (to reduce harm to zero), effectiveness (to demonstrate clinical outcomes) and experience (to deliver an excellent experience)'*. These priorities are upheld and maintained by the hospital's staff. Regular monitoring of clinical outcomes and the patient experience informs future improvements and changes for the benefit of the hospital's patients. Thus the hospital's values are enacted by the staff every day. The public are given a unique insight into what goes on behind the scenes through a popular television documentary series, which follows the lives of several patients from admission through treatment to discharge. GOSH has succeeded in building powerful positive perceptions amongst the general public and continues to do so, not only through clinical outcomes but also through a combination of strongly held values, sound priorities and effective, sensitive promotion.

Charles Mayo founded the Mayo Clinic (www.mayoclinic.org) in the USA in 1928, and since then it has grown to become internationally renowned, not only for its pioneering research and clinical care but also for building lasting, mutually beneficial relationships with a wide range of individuals and organizations. The clinic claims that its unique strength lies in its ability to *'take what some say can't be done and make it the new standard'*, which succinctly defines the clinic's mission. The clinic strives to get to know its patients and their needs so that they can deliver the sort of care that is most needed. It works closely with insurance companies, has created an advertising-free social network and offers patients eConsults. Building positive relationships is key to this service provider's success, as is an emphasis on the fact that the organization is not-for-profit, striving to deliver quality healthcare that is affordable. The Mayo Clinic actively seeks patients' and staff views and encourages comments from the general public. In this way, patients, staff and the public have a say in what the Mayo Clinic does and how it does it.

Approaches to branding in SMEs

Most veterinary hospitals in the UK are small to medium-sized businesses and, as such, may lack the marketing resources of larger organizations. A significant number are owned and managed by veterinary surgeons, and decision-making is centred around or controlled by individuals or small management teams. Berthon *et al.* (2008) observe that SMEs often face resource constraints, in terms of time and money, which leads many owner-managers to adopt a 'survival mentality'. However, SMEs, because they are smaller, can often be more innovative and more flexible in responding to changing customer needs. These factors influence the choice of branding strategy adopted by SMEs, and could potentially act as constraints when implementing a corporate branding approach, which often requires organization-wide change and additional resources.

Wong and Merrilees (2005) studied a range of Australian service SMEs and found that their interpretation of the brand concept was narrow, with implementation restricted to brand name, logo and advertising. Advertising on television, in Yellow Pages and via promotional leaflets was considered by these companies as less effective than personal selling or face-to-face communication with customers – strategies on which they relied heavily. They considered branding to be the preserve of large organizations and too expensive a marketing tool for their budgets. The paper's executive summary argued that these firms were misguided, because regardless of whether they sought to actively develop a brand or not, the 'unintentional' brand would inevitably emerge through the development of customers' opinions of their products. The disadvantage these firms had is that they were competing with branded organizations, which had actively managed their brands, and this had led to increased profits. The authors suggested that one way of making branding more accessible to these organizations was to 'rephrase' the brand concept so that it was more familiar to the entrepreneur – for example, by including such terms as reputation, quality, image, customer attitude and customer association. Thus branding for the smaller business would be based around four key activities:

- investing in the brand without sacrificing the direct sales effort, which is crucial to the smaller business;
- striving to be different and making sure customers know it;
- developing an internal culture where employees become brand advocates;
- consistent communications – defining the message and keeping it consistent.

Brand creation may indeed happen without any conscious effort on the part of the company – customers will inevitably develop an opinion about the product and the company simply through buying and using the products. So, a veterinary hospital need not do very much at all and its brand will emerge. However, this process is uncontrolled and may have undesirable or unwanted results. It is far better to actively build the brand in order to ensure that the associations formed by customers are those that the hospital intends. Also, developing a brand need not require a great deal of money or expense. By attending to the key basic concepts, a great deal can be achieved without expensive marketing.

Krake (2005) studied medium-sized companies in the Netherlands engaged in producing consumer goods. Although not relevant to services branding, his findings agreed in essence with those of Wong and Merrilees (2005) – entrepreneurs did not clearly understand brand management and did not see it as a priority for them. Few of the companies had a marketing manager and, consequently, the owners made most of the marketing decisions themselves. What was significant, however, was the key role played by the entrepreneur who utilized public relations activities in order to develop and promote the company name and image. Two things are relevant here: the need for greater understanding of branding strategies amongst business owners and the crucial role of the entrepreneur in delivering the message and creating the brand.

According to Merrilees (2007), the corporate branding strategy can provide an overarching, integrating tool for the entire process of new venture creation. It can support a range of functions, such as securing capital, increasing new customer acquisition and access to suppliers, amongst others. The role of the entrepreneur, again, emerges here as being key to promoting the brand.

Spence and Hamzaoui Essoussi (2010) observed that successful SME brands demonstrate core values of quality and innovation from the start, and these remain and are nurtured as the business grows. The firms they studied tended to differentiate their brands based on image, reputation and quality, amongst others. They used targeted media, in keeping with the characteristics of their customers, and well-designed websites, which supported the positioning of their brands.

If we now relate the findings discussed so far to veterinary hospitals as service-based SMEs, a number of useful observations can be made, as follows:

- Veterinary hospitals may need to adapt their branding strategies to take account of the availability of financial and physical resources. However, a great deal can be accomplished even with limited resources, provided the key basic branding principles, which have been outlined here, are adhered to.
- The role of the owner-manager in developing and promoting the brand is key, and that person acts as a 'brand champion' for the firm. It would be prudent for veterinary hospital owners and managers to identify a 'brand champion' early in the process. A suitable person may be chosen from amongst the management team or may need to be recruited from outside the hospital.
- The corporate branding approach can support the development of new enterprises by providing a framework for the management of necessary processes, communications and attitudes that would support the brand.
- Veterinary hospitals should ensure that they put in place methods of measuring the effectiveness of brand strategies; otherwise they will not be able to reliably assess the results of these strategies.

A proposed model for developing a veterinary hospital brand

De Chernatony et al. (2003) examined the process of building a services brand in order to identify and describe a development model. They carried out in-depth interviews with leading brand consultants to establish whether distinct stages in the process could be identified. A recurring consultant recommendation was that each stage should maintain a balanced internal and external orientation, giving equal attention to both internal processes and to the external customer experience. De Chernatony et al. (2003) propose a nine-stage development model. Davis (2002) proposes a four-phase 'brand asset management' model which includes a number of stages within each phase. This model claims to adopt a balanced orientation as recommended by the brand consultants in de Chernatony et al.'s (2003) study. The four phases of Davis's (2002) model happen to neatly map across to the model for building a corporate brand developed by Gregory and Sellers (2002). Davis's (2002) and

Table 8.2 Building a services brand

Davis (2002)	Gregory and Sellers (2002)
Phase 1: Develop a brand vision	1. Gather intelligence – build knowledge about the desired corporate brand
Phase 2: Determine the brand picture	2. Define the essence of the corporate brand (strategy phase)
Phase 3: Devise and agree a brand management strategy	3. Express the brand – for internal and external audiences
Phase 4: Devise a supporting culture	4. Gain staff commitment and build the infrastructure to support delivery of the brand (management phase)

Source: Adapted from Davis (2002) and Gregory and Sellers (2002).

Gregory and Sellers' (2002) models and their stages are summarized in Table 8.2.

Both models provide a useful starting point for considering a brand-building model suitable for implementation within a veterinary hospital. Drawing on this work, a seven-stage model for the implementation of a veterinary hospital brand is therefore proposed:

Stage 1: conduct an analysis of the hospital in order to: (1) identify current internal strengths and weaknesses (2) assess the opportunities and threats posed by the external environment within which the hospital operates.

This is known as a SWOT analysis. Close and honest scrutiny of what is and is not currently working is essential. A good way of finding this out is to gather opinions from staff and from clients about the service provided and about how they view the hospital. Customer satisfaction surveys are useful in obtaining current satisfaction ratings. The SWOT analysis should result in the identification of the hospital's specific competences, which can be developed further. Some services currently being offered may need to be discontinued in favour of a different package. This carries a greater risk, but may bring the desired level of differentiation from the services offered by direct competitors. The SWOT analysis should begin to clarify the sort of identity and values that the hospital wishes to espouse.

Stage 2: agree a brand vision. This involves finding the answers to the following key questions:

○ What are the hospital's values and what does the hospital stand for?
○ What does the hospital currently offer that is unique and that can be developed into a brand?
○ How can the brand essence be expressed in terms of a mission statement?

Clarification of brand values may mean a rethink of the hospital's client base, because some existing client groups and their needs may not fit with the new brand. The hospital will also consider at this stage whether it has the human and physical resources needed to implement the desired brand vision.

Stage 3: agree brand positioning. In other words, ensure that the hospital brand is sufficiently unique and that it provides real, honest value that can be trusted. This involves defining the core service or services, the methods of delivery and the prices to be charged.

Stage 4: communicate the hospital brand concept to all staff and gain their commitment to it. An effective way of achieving staff buy-in is to involve them from the outset in creating the hospital's vision and formulating its values, which should be summarized succinctly in a few key phrases, pinned up on notice boards around the hospital and repeated on corporate literature and on the hospital's website. It is essential that staff identify with and 'own' the brand. If they are unable to do so, they will be unable to deliver it consistently to clients.

Stage 5: ensure that all of the hospital's resources are in place to support the development of the brand. These resources include staff skills and attitudes, premises and equipment, procedures and protocols and, above all, clinical competence, transparency and accountability. Methods of monitoring all clinical outcomes should be put in place, as should client communication protocols.

Stage 6: promote the brand to clients and test it before rolling it out to all. All the external symbols of the brand, e.g. hospital name, logo, waiting room, corporate stationery, staff uniforms and client communication tools, will need to be redesigned to reflect the brand concept so that it is clearly recognizable by clients in everything they see and experience.

Stage 7: communicate and deliver a strong brand message consistently. A part of this is keeping one's promises. The processes by which the service is delivered are an integral part of the brand and so these must be continuously monitored to ensure that the brand vision and values are being delivered, and that the client experience is consistently positive, irrespective of whether the animal gets better or not.

The above stages are not meant to be strictly sequential. Clearly, some or all of the stages can be implemented concurrently. Finally, as has already been shown, success is more likely if there is a 'champion' capable of enthusing staff and keeping everyone motivated during the early stages of the process. This role could potentially be performed by the hospital director, hospital manager or by members of the team tasked with implementing the brand strategy.

Conclusions

Corporate branding is a holistic marketing approach, which is not only suitable for service-based business, but which can be utilized to create a veterinary hospital corporate brand. Whether hospital owners and managers choose to follow the structured approach, as outlined in this chapter, or whether they prefer a more informal approach, the process will inevitably lead to a rethink of the overall values the hospital represents and the image it wants to portray to its clients and others. A scrutiny of internal processes and procedures and the way the service is delivered to clients is a likely consequence of the corporate branding approach.

It is arguable whether veterinary hospitals can continue to thrive in the current economic climate without considerable marketing effort to ensure competitiveness, but it is through the quality of its services, premises and equipment, but particularly its staff, that real value is delivered to clients. Branding merely helps clients to see this value more clearly.

Summary

This chapter has drawn on a range of published sources to explain the brand concept. It has defined and discussed three key dimensions of branding: brand identity, brand values and brand equity. These concepts have been explored in the context of service based SMEs and the veterinary sector. A model for developing a veterinary hospital brand has also been presented.

Review questions

1. Give an example of a branded product (or service) with which you are familiar, and describe the brand values represented by this product (or service).
2. Discuss the specific challenges marketers face when marketing services as opposed to products.
3. Explain why the corporate branding approach is an appropriate marketing strategy for veterinary services.
4. In what ways can branding give a veterinary hospital an advantage over its competitors?
5. Give at least four reasons why staff are crucial to the delivery of the brand in service-based businesses.

Acknowledgements

Reproduced with permission from 'The Veterinary Nurse': Coates CR (2013) Building a veterinary practice brand. The Veterinary Nurse 4 (2): in press.

References

Aaker, D.A., 1996. Building Strong Brands. Free Press/Simon & Schuster, New York.

Berry, L.L., 2000. Cultivating service brand equity. Journal of the Academy of Marketing Science 28 (1), 128–137.

Berthon, P., Hulbert, J., Pitt, L.F., 1999. Brand management prognostications. Sloan Manage. Rev. Winter, 53–64.

Berthon, P., Ewing, M.T., Napoli, J., 2008. Brand management in small to medium-sized enterprises. Journal of Small Business Management 46 (1), 27–45.

Dall'Olmo, F., de Chernatony, L., 2000. The service brand as relationships builder. British Journal of Management 11, 137–150.

Davidson, H., 1997. Even More Offensive Marketing. Penguin Books, London.

Davis, S., 2002. Implementing your BAM strategy: 11 steps to making your brand a more valuable business asset. Journal of Consumer Marketing 19 (6), 503–513.

De Chernatony, L., Segal-Horn, S., 2001. Building on services' characteristics to develop successful services brands. Journal of Marketing Management 17, 645–669.

De Chernatony, L., Dall'Olmo Riley, F., 1999. Experts' views about defining services brands and the principles of services branding. Journal of Business Research 46, 181–192.

De Chernatony, L., Drury, S., Segal-Horn, S., 2003. Building a services brand: stages, people and orientations. Service Industries Journal 23 (3), 1–21.

Feldwick, P., 1996. Do we really need 'brand equity'? Journal of Brand Management 4 (1), 9–28.

Gregory, J., Sellers, L.J., 2002. Building corporate brands. Pharmaceutical Executive 22 (1), 38–44.

Jobber, D., 2001. Principles and Practice of Marketing, third ed. McGraw-Hill, Maidenhead, UK.

Keller, K.L., Lehmann, D.R., 2006. Brands and branding: research findings and future priorities. Marketing Science 25 (6), 740–759.

Krake, F.B.G.J.M., 2005. Successful brand management in SMEs: a new theory and practical hints. Journal of Product and Brand Management 14 (4), 228–238.

Merrilees, B., 2007. A theory of brand-led SME new venture development. Qualitative Market Research 10 (4), 403–415.

Pringle, H., Gordon, W., 2001. Brand Manners: How to Create the Self-Confident Organization to Live the Brand. Wiley, Chichester, UK.

Spence, M., Hamzaoui Essoussi, L., 2010. SME brand building and management: an exploratory study. European Journal of Marketing 44 (7/8), 1037–1054.

Wong, H.Y., Merrilees, B., 2005. A brand orientation typology for SMEs: a case research approach. Journal of Product and Brand Management 14 (3), 155–162.

Wood, L., 2000. Brands and brand equity: definition and management. Management Decision 38 (9), 662–669.

Veterinary field expertise and knowledge exchange

9

Jeremy Phillipson   Amy Proctor   Philip Lowe
Andrew Donaldson

CHAPTER OVERVIEW

Veterinary practices are examples of knowledge-intensive business services, i.e. businesses that rely heavily on the high-quality clinical and technical skills of those they employ. This is, in fact, their key business asset: the way they market and deploy this asset is the foundation of their effective performance, and the way they nurture and renew it is fundamental to their future. In exploring contemporary challenges in veterinary business management, understanding the fundamental processes by which veterinarians develop their knowledge and pass this on is critical for effective professional practice and for the broader promotion of a knowledge-based economy. At a time when the large-animal veterinary sector is under pressure to reassert its importance within the profession, this chapter explores the ways in which food animal veterinarians keep their knowledge of livestock health and production up to date in practice, and considers how this knowledge could be used to secure the role of the veterinarian in the future. While the chapter focuses on farm animal veterinarians as a case study, many of the issues raised here have wider applicability to veterinarians working in companion and equine fields, including the key themes of knowledge renewal and on-the-job learning, inter-professional working and the veterinarian as a key agent of knowledge exchange.

LEARNING OUTCOMES

After reading this chapter, students will be able to:
- Understand the key ways in which veterinarians maintain and renew their knowledge once in practice.
- Appreciate the contribution of experiential and experimental knowledge derived from on-the-job learning to veterinary expertise.
- Understand how interaction with veterinary colleagues, clients and other professionals contributes to the development of veterinary knowledge and expertise
- Realize that veterinarians have a key role to play as knowledge brokers within the agri-food system.
- Recognize the importance of veterinarians understanding the value of their knowledge and their potential brokerage role as a marketable product within the veterinary business.

Introduction

Farm animal veterinarians are part of the knowledge-based economy in which professionals earn their livelihood by selling their expertise directly to clients. They play a key role in enhancing the skills and development of tens of thousands of farming businesses, and are required to keep their knowledge up to date in practice, as they face complex and ever-changing calls on their expertise. According to the standard formulation of knowledge transfer, 'field professionals' such as farm animal veterinary surgeons (but also agronomists, nutritionists, ecologists, etc.) act as intermediaries bringing science to the farm. In addition, veterinarians broker different types of knowledge apart from formal science. They also generate new knowledge and actively solve problems that they encounter as they strive to safeguard animal and public health. Veterinarians build

© 2014, Elsevier Ltd.

up their own experiential and experimental knowledge in and through practice. They are not simply transferors of knowledge from others, but combine, translate and repackage information, and draw on their own accumulated field knowledge to tailor it to the circumstances of the client. Veterinarians thus act as both agents of knowledge exchange and practical problem solvers. To equip them for these roles, and to facilitate more effective knowledge exchange strategies, it is vital that new graduates not only have a clear understanding of these everyday knowledge practices, but also understand their wider significance as a valuable asset and marketable product in an increasingly competitive business environment.

The chapter is structured as follows. First, we examine the underpinning knowledge systems of veterinarians before exploring the processes through which this knowledge is formed and renewed, with a particular focus on the importance of field-generated knowledge. We then consider what veterinarians gain in terms of on-the-job learning from their interactions with colleagues, clients and other professionals. We conclude by exploring the role of practising veterinarians in knowledge exchange strategies for animal and public health, and consider how their field-generated knowledge could prove critical to securing their role in the future.

This chapter reflects on recent research carried out by the authors exploring the composition of field expertise and the role of farm advisors in knowledge exchange. 'Science in the field: understanding the changing role of expertise in the rural economy' was an Economic and Social Research Council-funded research project which ran between 2008 and 2011, and investigated how farm advisors such as land agents, vets and ecologists could be an important link in bridging the gap between scientific research and land management practice. The project involved in-depth face-to-face interviews with advisors, their professional associations and farmers, as well as ethnographic work, including work-shadowing of advisors going about their day-to-day work and observation of training and professional development activities. We present the findings from this research in the form of direct quotes taken from the interviews. All quotes used in the text are from interviews with practising veterinarians unless otherwise stated (these have been anonymized to maintain confidentiality).

The knowledge systems of field veterinarians

The Foresight Report on the future of food and farming in the UK identified the improvement of advisory services to farmers, land managers and food producers as a top priority in tackling the challenges of food security (Foresight, 2010, 2011). Changing commercial and legislative pressures on farmers create a need for up-to-date professional advice. However, concerns have been raised over the capacity of the agricultural advisory system to incorporate the latest insights from science (Oreszczyn et al., 2010; Van Crowder and Anderson, 1997). In animal husbandry, the requirement to increase productivity, while at the same time protecting the environment and animal welfare, necessitates continuous improvements in the skills and knowledge applied to livestock management under veterinary advice and direction. Furthermore, as government hands over more of the responsibility for managing animal health and disease risk to the agricultural industry, vets have to rethink the services they provide to their customers. Veterinary work can be conceptualized as a suite of services for livestock and food producers, including knowledge transfer, evaluation and planning. Knowledge management and getting expert advice to where it is needed are absolutely critical to the effectiveness of risk management and responsibility sharing. The new external challenges facing farming and food production (e.g. climate change, potential shifts in disease patterns, economic and energy concerns, and an emerging policy focus on food supply and risk) place a premium on knowledge that is up to date, authoritative, practical and targeted. Veterinary graduates qualify with an impressive knowledge and skill set, but there are questions concerning the extent to which professional and lifelong learning skills are integrated into the curriculum (May, 2008). In this chapter we explore how veterinarians maintain their knowledge, skills and expertise once their formal training has concluded and they enter professional practice.

When asked what formal knowledge updates they need to draw on in their work, vets refer not just to scientific knowledge but also to professional knowledge, such as that concerning professional standards and conduct, and regulatory knowledge, concerning policy or guidance documents, and new legislation impacting the profession (as illustrated in the right-hand side of Figure 9.1).

Professional associations are the most important source of all three types of formal knowledge.

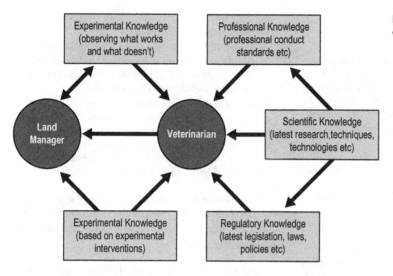

Figure 9.1 • The nature of veterinarians' field expertise

Practising vets expect their professional associations to filter out and synthesize scientific and regulatory developments relevant to their work. The professional channels used for knowledge updating include programmed continuing professional development (CPD), websites, publications, conferences, events and meetings of specialist divisions. Veterinarians also update their knowledge through other channels including training and information provided in-house or by sectoral bodies like the National Farmers' Union, the Agricultural and Horticulture Development Board (via levy bodies like EBLEX, the organization for the English beef and sheep meat industry, and BPEX, the organization representing pig levy payers in England), and through private companies, particularly veterinary pharmaceutical firms. Books, journals, magazines, circulars and the farming press are also important as key knowledge sources, as is the Internet (via reference sites such as PubMed).

The formal professional, regulatory and scientific sources veterinarians draw upon do not, however, fully reflect the range of ways they keep their expertise up to date and problem-solve. Advisors actively broker a range of different types of knowledge, besides formal science, including generating knowledge themselves through learning on the job. For veterinarians, great significance is placed on this field-generated knowledge (see the left-hand side of Figure 9.1). Therefore, we need to rethink traditional understandings of their role as simply intermediaries of formal knowledge.

The significance of field-generated knowledge

As agents of knowledge exchange, veterinarians relay information and expertise to farmers, much of which is drawn from professional, regulatory and scientific sources. However, veterinarians are not simply transferors to their clients of formal knowledge from scientists or other experts; they are also agents of knowledge application, adaptation and practical problem solvers. As a result, they are able to produce interactively distinctive and specialized field knowledge. Veterinarians' field knowledge comprises both experiential and experimental knowledge. Experiential and experimental knowledge are derived from observation and intervention in practice; they are related in that they both stem from 'direct experience' (Fazey *et al.*, 2006). These forms of knowledge become implicit through an 'intuitive process, based on substantial, long-term and reflected experience' (Baars, 2011, p. 602).

Experiential knowledge involves learning through personal observation of what works and what does not. It is expertise derived from example and trial and error, and is refined through replication and iteration, case by case. It is, essentially, learning about what works in specific contexts, often intuitively so, and is seen by practitioners as crucial to the formation and renewal of field expertise. Some veterinarians described, for example, how they learnt from the mistakes they had made in the early years on entering practice:

> There's no doubt that the practical experiences you get are absolutely vital to temper your advice, and as much as anything to know what harm you can do with advice and it's very possible to improve one thing and make another thing a lot worse, and it's that kind of whole farm context and experience of things going wrong probably that is the most important thing.

> Different conditions occur in different localities, certain things that I'd never have seen in Scotland, or where I saw practice, but here they're very common things. It gets done, you know, you make the mistakes and you don't recognize certain things, you speak to your colleagues, other people in the locality, work it out, but once you've got it you've got it.

In interview, veterinarians described how they also learnt through replication and refinement of different techniques and approaches:

> Your progression is [down to] experience; it's cases and doing things for the second, third, fourth time – seeing things.

> It is always the easiest way to recognize, diagnose, and treat something if you've seen it before. So the first time you see something you don't know to what degree it's abnormal, to what degree it's going to respond to X, Y, or Z, but if you've been there before you've got something to relate back to, you remember it well, and you know how it's going to go.

> It's the sort of job that constantly pushes you anyway. It constantly pushes your knowledge, so you'll see a case, you'll have found out what it was, so you see another one next time and you'll go, 'Ah, I know what that is. We did this last time; the prognosis is poor based on the last case.'

> We are trained to think as a scientist and to question and to rely on evidence as much as we can. Obviously there are areas of the jigsaw that aren't filled in and we have to therefore use experience. Experience is when it's worked for you twice, you think that's the way to do it. You're continually valuating your experience against the science and then you're interpreting this in the light of the problem that's facing you.

In addition, veterinarians also utilize a different source of field knowledge – experimental knowledge – generated through deliberate interventions in the field. This experimental knowledge derives from problem solving, with veterinarians systematically trying out different approaches. Vets try things out in a range of different ways. In our study, this included, for example, informal investigations involving the fieldwork of testing, observing and monitoring:

> We do in-house research; it's not ground breaking ... for example this year we've been involved in a foot bathing

trial for a sheep foot bath, which wasn't high science that was just in-practice style research.

> ... periodically you will try something slightly less routine, by way of just modifying the treatment or incorporating copper sulphate into a foot pressing or something else like that, which is slightly outwith the norm.

> None of it is particularly scientific, but on-farm trials mainly just doing something and assessing the effect and hopefully measuring and weighing and reporting things. Obviously we can't do anything scientific in the sense that as soon as you get into anything like sampling and what-not, we need home office licences.

Veterinarians also described a range of experimental activity. Much of this involved informal experimentation such as approaches and attitudes to administering drugs:

> You play around with dose rates, different drugs ... there are lots of different ways to skin a cat as it were. I had to go and castrate a reindeer last week, which is all brand new to me, so that was pretty much experimental working out the dose rate.

> A lot of things are a little bit experiment-wise in terms of, you know, a batch of sick lambs or something and I'll go, 'Right, I'll give those five that kind of antibiotic, those five that kind, and those five that kind,' and see which ones live, see how they do. And there's a bit of doing things cheap ... there was a farm with a big worm burden and we were worried about worming resistance so I wanted to go in and do a test. It was the wrong time of year and we came to an agreement that we'll do it cheap and if it doesn't work because it was the wrong time of year, it was the wrong type of sheep, it'll be free, and if it does work you'll pay for it but at a reduced level.

> I mean, most cases are an experiment, you put the drugs in and you see what happens, but you have a wee bit of a diagnosis, a bit of an idea ... we do a lot of blood sampling of sheep, in particular, for trace elements ... we take lots of faecal samples looking for worm burdens.

In interview, some veterinarians recounted cases where they had even modified surgical techniques as part of their experimentation:

> A particular example that we've been doing recently is auditing some of our surgery that we do on the cattle side – caesareans and displaced stomach operations, auditing the success of those. Obviously we then look at that and make decisions as to whether there are changes that we should make in technique or approach or sterilization or whatever.

> Surgery, in terms of experimentation, you just modify your technique from one to another, or as the case dictates. But on the medicine side of things, you're very largely restricted if you play things by the book.

> ... part of what keeps the job fresh is if you become aware of a technique for solving a certain problem, then it's quite

refreshing that you can actually try it and see how it goes ... there are several different ways to perform just about every surgical technique that there is, and you can give them a try. We've still got that flexibility with our clients to do that.

Some veterinarians also described more formal types of experimentation, including participating in clinical trials and contributing towards drug company research:

> We do a bit of work for [a pharmaceutical company] – drug trials, that sort of thing. That's quite lucrative. Since the recession that seems to have just fallen on its head. We've done a bit of trial work for ... another drug company. Again, they've supplied the drugs and maybe the lab fees and we've done the visits, and the injecting, and the follow-up.

In these ways, veterinarians in the field use their experience and knowledge to develop systematic approaches to individual cases. There are limits to how far veterinarians can experiment due to restrictions of drug licences, costs and clients' attitudes. It is also recognized that, owing to its often informal nature, such experimentation lacks rigour, such as not using control groups. Nevertheless, practitioners value experimentation as a means to extend their knowledge, address gaps in their formal knowledge/training, test their skills and solve problems. They also understand what would be needed to turn this field experimentation into 'proper research', as one veterinarian explained:

> We found a worm that was resistant to wormer in hill sheep, which is really rare. And it got even the serious sheep bods at the Research Institute quite excited. So I did write that up for a presentation to other vets on a CPD evening. We did each animal with something different and took samples before and after ... Everything wasn't absolutely up to the knocker but I got a result, and that ties in with what was going on with the farmer. That farm has now changed its worming strategy. And I was able to have something to present to other sheep vets and it raised a lot of questions.

Learning through interaction with others

Field knowledge is not simply self-generated; it derives from interactions with others. In our study, veterinarians emphasized the importance of learning from colleagues, from clients and from other professionals (via inter-professional working) where they were found to exchange different types of knowledge and generate new expertise. Field knowledge is therefore a combination of experiential (reflective), experimental and interpersonal skills.

Veterinary colleagues

Our findings showed that advisors from within the same profession often share experiences and pass on 'best practice'. Skills are learnt through interaction with other, more experienced practitioners who can demonstrate, guide and give feedback on what should be done. For veterinarians, colleagues may share knowledge and expertise via informal discussion back at the practice, or formal mentoring out in the field:

> As a new grad ... if you're having difficulty at 1 a.m. in the morning with a difficult case, being able to ring someone and say, 'Can you come and help me?' And rather than getting, 'No, piss off, get yourself sorted out, just get on with it,' someone going, 'Yeah, no worries, I'll come out and give you a hand.' I suppose that's more support than teamwork isn't it? But that's very much needed, because it is experience-based learning. So that makes a difference.

Other veterinarians explained how they had learnt from the good practice of colleagues, sometimes from direct observation and other times from indirect accounts relayed to them:

> You are literally just sort of thrown into firsthand practice, and that is why veterinary new grads tend to either sink or swim, depending on whether the practice is supportive. This practice, I did work experience as a student here. I'd maybe done four or five [cow caesareans] during normal hours with someone helping me, and then took the plunge and did one out of hours, and that was the first one. If it's something particularly difficult surgery wise, we would try and take two vets out onto the farm. So my first fertility testing, that sort of thing, there would be two vets going out.
>
> When I first graduated, I used to ring guys that I saw practice with and ask 'What the bloody hell do I do with this?' and they would laugh down the phone and say 'Try this.' Sometimes it worked, sometimes it didn't. It's not like you are going back to your boss, the guy who is paying you the money, and going 'I don't know what to do.'

When veterinarians encounter an unfamiliar problem that they are unable to resolve by consulting immediate colleagues, they are likely to seek advice from personal contacts in veterinary colleges, laboratories or pharmaceutical companies. These informal sources, which include contacts developed during formal training and through professional networks, are therefore crucial for maintaining and renewing scientific knowledge. There are also occasions of a reversal in knowledge flows, with many veterinarians referring to the role of placement veterinary students or recent graduates in passing on the latest research to established practitioners in the field.

Clients

As agents of knowledge exchange, veterinarians often assume a training/didactic role with clients, relaying expertise and information:

> Fewer and fewer farmers seem to want to just present you with a sick cow or a problem, and you just make it go away without their engagement, so they want to understand, they are becoming more and more technically competent, and they have a relatively limited number of avenues for getting that increase in technical knowledge, and the veterinarian has got to be an important part of that.

Alongside this training mode, veterinarians may also assume a problem-solving role, often in conjunction with their clients. Veterinarians test out their experimental knowledge on farmers, and also develop experiential knowledge through their interactions with them. This joint learning alongside clients was acknowledged, with veterinarian and farmer working together, handling the animals, exchanging their knowledge and experience of different issues and discussing responses to problems *in situ*. This included, for example, veterinarians and farmers debating different drug options and treatments; discussing a particular animal's medical history; evaluating whether certain animals might require a caesarean and when the best time might be to perform this; and making assessments of the suitability of different animals for breeding purposes.

> A lot of farmers, stockmen, owners, whatever, will have innovative ideas every now and again, or they'll have heard something from either a meeting that we haven't been to or from a friend of theirs or they've read or whatever, and we will evaluate that ...Taking knowledge from them, we do do that, there's no doubt about it. I'm sometimes not wanting to shout it from the rooftops because they'll think, 'Well, you pay us, then.'

Veterinarians also learn a lot from their clients about the business of farming and their knowledge of husbandry and land management:

> It's a two-way discussion because they've got loads of knowledge that you can learn from. I suppose if you're talking purely about mastitis then they're probably not

going to give as much as you can give. But things like nutrition and housing ... definitely.

> It's amazing how much you learn ... broadening your knowledge of the industry, talking to clients. You can go through the price of grain, the price of fat cattle, the price of store lambs in that 40 minutes of having a cup of tea.

> Well, a lot of them know a lot about the ancillary sides of things, so they know a lot about the mechanics of farming or the housing or how things work, and some know a lot about ventilation, some don't, some know a lot about feeding systems, etc.

Such knowledge was regarded as vital to helping veterinarians understand the practical and commercial context into which their technical advice must fit. This combining of knowledge – which might include elements of agronomy, animal husbandry, farm economics, disease ecology and livestock geography – is also vital to veterinarians' understanding of their local and regional context. In conveying advice, veterinarians will also take into consideration factors such as the social context and aspirations of the farmer and their families, as well as the technical capabilities and commercial objectives of the farm business. The art of communication and building a rapport and relationship with clients are crucial factors in determining how much knowledge exchange takes place between veterinarian and farmer. This is increasingly recognized within veterinary schools with the introduction of communications skills into the professional skills elements.

Other professionals

The knowledge veterinarians obtain from working with other field-based professionals is becoming increasingly significant. Until the early 1990s, responsibility for knowledge transfer in farming was largely assumed by government in the form of state-funded agricultural extension (Dancey, 1993; Jones and Garforth, 1997; Leeuwis and Van den Ban, 2004; Rivera and Sulaiman, 2009; Swanson *et al.*, 1997). The privatization of agricultural extension and the consequent restructuring of extension services involved a major switch in the philosophy of knowledge production and delivery, from one based on a 'top-down' model of science application and technological diffusion to one oriented to the knowledge needs, agency and indigenous expertise of the client. In this more open market for field knowledge there has also been a proliferation and fragmentation of knowledge providers. One of the fears associated with the privatization of extension services was that agricultural knowledge provision would be compartmentalized into a series of closed systems, with a 'decrease in information which is openly exchanged on a free-of-charge basis among various actors' (Klerkx *et al.*, 2006, p. 191). In fact, the contemporary advisory landscape is characterized by a pluralistic system of field advisors – a mixed economy of expertise. The shift towards pluralistic extension systems involving a range of specialized actors is significant; veterinarians need to have an understanding of the contemporary advisory landscape within which they operate. Crucially, they need to be able to negotiate their way across expert divides in order to exchange and access knowledge.

Advisors from different professions are increasingly required to collaborate on behalf of clients, exchanging different types of knowledge and generating new expertise. For veterinarians, this inter-professional working may involve feed advisors, nutritionists, artificial insemination technicians, foot trimmers/farriers, animal housing/design consultants as well as pharmaceutical company representatives. These advisory collaborations serve not only as a platform for a one-way flow of information (e.g. when an advisor is providing advice to a farmer) but also for the negotiation of knowledge and authority between different advisors. In their dealings with some other professionals, veterinarians acknowledge complementary relations and assert the value of teamwork:

> I find the people that are very useful are the drug reps, or the vets that actually work for the drug companies, they're very useful on the use of drugs from their own past experiences. It's really good to get friendly with them, they're a good mine of information and generally in that job they do a lot of speaking and presenting, they're pretty good communicators. It's their job to communicate with the likes of me so it's not like you're bugging them, that's what they're there for.

> Lameness in sheep and dairy cattle is a major problem. If it's a recognizable problem, then we go out of our way to become involved with a foot trimmer. Apart from anything else, you can shortcut an awful lot of dead-end approaches by checking through the foot trimmer's records.

> One of our dairy clients was having a lot of trouble with cows with cysts. It happened to be a farm that myself and Sarah, one of the vets, were in charge of. The farmer said how he was getting his nutritionist to come in. I couldn't attend, so I said to Sarah, 'He's got the nutritionist coming. We should be there because it's a team effort to try and get this problem resolved. Sarah was quite alarmed, because we did nutrition in first and second year. She's been eight years qualified, so it's eleven years ago, and she didn't feel confident to be involved in that

discussion with the nutritionist. I said, 'Well, you don't need to know about nutrition. You just need to know about the physiology of the cyst, we've still got tonight to read up about it, so you can turn up tomorrow morning and you're going to know all about cysts. You'll have something to contribute. Not only that, you'll absorb some of the nutritional information from the nutritionist. The farmer can see that we're keen to work as a team with his other advisors, we'll learn something from it, the nutritionist will probably learn something from us, and everybody is better off.' So she came back. 'How did you get on?' 'It was marvellous.' Now she knows that the next time the same thing happens with another farm, at least she can go in with knowledge about the physiology of a cyst, plus a little bit of nutrition.

With other professionals, veterinarians may develop a more competitive relationship. This might require them to assert more control or authority over a situation:

> I'm thinking of a food advisor I work with; I don't find him easy, I think he's quite nervous when he's around me, but he's got his laptop and he can put a ration together and it'll be fine. He never goes out and watches the cows, he does that without leaving the farmer's kitchen, now that's wrong, and that's why he and I go out for a farm walk every now and again and we look at the condition of the cows and the condition of the concrete and the tracks and all that kind of stuff.

In such situations, understanding both the limits of their own and others' expertise is crucial for effective inter-professional working:

> I actually have on my laptop scanned in all the sheets from the last visit of the foot trimmer to the farm, we're looking for patterns of disease; we can work together like that. It's a team thing but it's limited, and the important thing is an understanding of what he can do and what he can't. He looked at the foot; he doesn't know what's going on in the rest of the animal. They have their place and then you work together. They spot there's a problem going on but then the veterinarian becomes linked into solving it.

Becoming an effective expert requires not only the specialist knowledge of your own field but also knowing how to position yourself in wider networks of advice and expertise. In some situations, veterinarians position themselves at the centre of overlapping networks, and assert their centrality by performing bridging roles between different specialists:

> There are lots of other sorts of advice, farm consultants and the like, who have an important role to play … but I think it's important that the vets make sure that our voices are heard as well.

> We had a case where there were some fairly catastrophic health problems on a dairy farm. We called in an external

nutritionist and he came along to try and address things. In that situation, by way of a goodwill gesture, we arrived to coordinate things and didn't charge for that time or visit.

These quotes highlight the significance of inter-professional working as a crucial part of the advisory process, but they also highlight some of the challenges. Operating as part of complex, multi-professional networks, veterinarians have to develop skills of negotiation and networking in order to navigate inter-professional competition and cooperation. This is how knowledge exchange occurs across different professions (Klerkx and Proctor, 2013). Cut off from the centralized certainty of state-managed extension, field advisors are now more reliant on each other. Their work is dependent on knowledge and skills beyond their own, and they have to develop skills in negotiating professional boundaries, including dealing with issues such as trust, teamwork and client relations (Proctor et al., 2012).

Strategies for improving recognition of veterinarians as knowledge brokers

Vets are key players in applying knowledge and expertise to livestock farming. As part of this, they act as intermediaries bringing science to farmers, but they are not mere conduits of formal science. As we have seen, they also broker different types of knowledge and generate new field knowledge of their own. As scientifically trained professionals and field-based practitioners, veterinarians derive and renew their expertise from both science and practice. However, this unorthodox creativity tends to be regarded with scepticism by veterinary academics and researchers:

> I know that every single thing that you do in practice is based on research because without that it would be hearsay, it would be hocus pocus.
>
> Research director

We're collecting data from veterinarians in the field to analyse, to give us the indications of that disease prevalence, etc. The issue coming back over and over again, for various people who we talked to about this, is that this isn't going to be very valid data, because it has been collected by veterinarians in the field and therefore it will be flawed ... It won't be as rigorous ... it won't be as robust in terms of categorization, diagnoses, whatever you want really, because it will have been collected by non-experts.

> Veterinary school scientist

Such views sit alongside an apparent lack of curiosity in veterinary schools towards experimental knowledge generated through practice, and reinforce a professional demarcation between researchers and practitioners. Students' main exposure to everyday veterinary work comes from the requirement for extramural studies. How field-generated knowledge is developed and its contribution to veterinary expertise has been given limited recognition by those responsible for training veterinarians and overseeing their professional development once in practice.

There is a parallel situation in human medicine. From interviews with Canadian clinicians, Mylopoulos and Scardamalia conclude that 'thus far, innovation in medicine has relied on a knowledge translation model ... emphasizing the ... incorporation of new research into daily practice. This exclusive emphasis has led to the devaluing of ideas generated through the daily innovative practice of health care workers for the purpose of practice-based, collaborative knowledge building' (Mylopoulos and Scardamalia, 2008, p. 980). In small-animal medicine, however, the potential seems to be more recognized, leading one commentator to claim that 'Practice-based clinical research is potentially a colossal resource for the veterinary profession. Much of the best veterinary clinical research has been produced by practitioners' (Holmes, 2009, p. 521).

Strategies must be developed to improve the authority of veterinary field expertise. The scale of field-based experiential and experimental learning suggests that veterinary schools may need to reconsider the type of skills that vets require to equip them throughout their professional careers. In reflecting on medical training, Mylopoulos and Regehr make the point that 'as they progress along the path towards becoming lifelong learners, students must be taught to recognize problem solving not only as a process of applying past knowledge, but also as an opportunity to produce and evolve new knowledge' (Mylopoulos and Regehr, 2009, p. 131). It is not clear to what extent veterinary schools see themselves as preparing such practical experimentalists, whether in terms of students' self-image or in terms of appropriate skills. Formal CPD provision and requirements do not fully capture the range of ways that practising vets keep their expertise up to date. Field-generated expertise, in particular, is not given its due recognition, and training provision does not seek to improve its rigour and authority. This is particularly important for knowledge exchange strategies which rely on the agency of vets (e.g. initiatives devised by government or dissemination and engagement strategies built into research programmes) as they need to be fully informed of the way veterinarians maintain their knowledge in the field.

Veterinary research agendas have become disconnected from technical dissemination capacities and vice versa. Working vets complain that they lack time to refresh their scientific knowledge. They consider that most scientific output (i.e. research published in academic journals) is not relevant or applicable to what they do. They express concerns about the shift in public funding away from applied work towards 'blue-sky' research. Veterinarians look to their professional bodies to filter the latest research findings and synthesize what scientific developments are relevant to their work, but this is unevenly done and professional associations are often marginal to public research decision-making. There is a need to improve knowledge exchange between the veterinary profession and the research base so that advisory services are better sensitized to the latest research and research is more responsive to the challenges of contemporary livestock farming.

Academic research institutions, programmes and projects could make better use of veterinarians in knowledge exchange. The Lowe report recommended that 'As the knowledge professionals in animal health, [vets] should be much more actively involved in the design and execution of programmes of research and knowledge management in animal disease and public health' (Lowe, 2009, p. 81). Farm animal veterinarians play a pivotal role at the interface of research and practice. In order to facilitate more effective knowledge exchange strategies it is vital that this role is first better recognized by all concerned; then knowledge transfer strategies that rely on veterinarians as intermediaries need to be better informed about their knowledge practices.

There are a number of organizations that carry out more applied, field-based 'development research' or 'near market' research into animal health and welfare matters such as EBLEX and the Scottish Agricultural College. These organizations often commission research projects which use practising vets for their local knowledge, technical support (i.e. collecting samples or data) and for recruiting farmers to studies. They also have dissemination strategies built into their projects which target vets to receive research outputs. One strategy for achieving stronger links between academic research and practice could involve the strengthening of links between research organizations and professional bodies – one of the key knowledge sources for veterinarians – to maximize knowledge exchange opportunities (Proctor et al., 2011).

Conclusions

Veterinarians are valued for the expertise they can bring to bear in helping clients overcome pressing problems and plan for future business development. For veterinary practices, as small businesses themselves, the maintenance and renewal of knowledge and expertise are vital to their functioning as competitive and successful enterprises. A key part of this requires the veterinary profession to understand and recognize that its brokerage role is crucial to its success. Farmers and animal keepers look to veterinarians to absorb complex, ambivalent messages and 'translate' them into terms they can understand. In conveying advice on animal health and welfare, vets will also take into consideration factors such as bio-security and the local ecology of disease, as well as the technical capabilities and commercial objectives of the farm business. Thus they do not simply transfer knowledge from other experts; they combine and repackage information and draw on their own accumulated field expertise in order to tailor the knowledge to the circumstances of the individual farmer. Above all, an experienced veterinarian knows what advice will work on a farm.

At a time when government is looking to farmers and industry to take on more of the costs and responsibility for animal disease and welfare, new leadership is needed beyond government and this is dependent upon the effective availability of good professional advice and expertise. To retain its influence, the profession needs to explore how it can capitalize on this shifting agenda. The profession will have to devise solutions that rely less on regulation and enforcement, and more on a collaborative approach and expert leadership. Veterinarians themselves undoubtedly need to become more consumer-centric, understanding the needs of their clients, and the markets into which farmers sell, to ensure they add value to the farm business and secure the custom of farmers. Veterinarians historically were a major influence on animal health policy because of their expertise; they could creatively engage again through a renewed attention to their field expertise (Enticott et al., 2011). Understanding the significance of their field-based knowledge and their role in brokering such knowledge as a valuable and marketable product is certainly one key way in which veterinarians can ensure they remain competitive as small businesses in this changing regulatory environment.

Summary

In examining the underpinning knowledge systems of veterinarians, this chapter has explored the processes whereby their knowledge is formed and renewed, with a particular focus on the importance of field-generated knowledge. In considering how this knowledge is then transferred and communicated, this chapter has explored the role that practising veterinarians play in knowledge exchange and how this role could be further developed to extract greater value for the veterinary business.

Review questions

1. What are the key ways in which farm veterinarians maintain and renew their scientific, professional and regulatory knowledge?

2. What are experiential and experimental knowledge, and how do veterinarians develop these?

3. Why should veterinarians be viewed as key knowledge brokers in the agri-food system?

4. Why should research institutions, programmes and projects make better use of veterinarians in knowledge exchange?

Acknowledgements

The research upon which this chapter is based was funded by the Economic and Social Research Council (RES 229-25-0025).

References

Baars, T., 2011. Experiential science; towards an integration of implicit and reflected practitioner-expert knowledge in the scientific development of organic farming. J. Agr. Environ. Ethics 24, 601–628.

Dancey, R.J., 1993. The evolution of agricultural extension in England and Wales. J. Agric. Econ. 44 (3), 375–393.

Enticott, G., Donaldson, A., Lowe, P., et al., 2011. The changing role of veterinary expertise in the food chain. Philosophical Transactions of the Royal Society B 366 (1573), 1955–1965.

Fazey, I., Fazey, J.A., Salisbury, J.G., Lindenmayer, D.B., Dovers, S., 2006. The nature and role of experiential knowledge for environmental conservation. Environ. Conserv. 33 (1), 1–10.

Foresight, 2010. Land Use Futures Project: Final Project Report. Government Office for Science, London.

Foresight, 2011. The Future of Food and Farming: Final Project Report. The Government Office for Science, London.

Holmes, M., 2009. Practice-based clinical research: an introduction. In Pract. 31, 520–523.

Jones, G.E., Garforth, C., 1997. The history, development, and future of agricultural extension. In:

Swanson, B.E., Bentz, R.P., Sofranko, A.J. (Eds.), Improving Agricultural Extension: A Reference Manual. FAO, Rome Chapter 1.

Klerkx, L., Proctor, A., 2013. Beyond fragmentation and disconnect: networks for knowledge exchange in the English land management advisory system. Land Use Policy 30, 13–24.

Klerkx, L., De Grip, K., Leeuwis, C., 2006. Hands off but strings attached: the contradictions of policy-induced demand-driven agricultural extension. Agr. Hum. Values 23, 189–204.

Leeuwis, C., Van den Ban, A., 2004. Communication for Rural Innovation: Rethinking Agricultural Extension. Blackwell, Oxford.

Lowe, P., 2009. Unlocking Potential: a Report on Veterinary Expertise in Food Animal Production. Report to the Vets and Veterinary Services Steering Group. DEFRA, London.

May, S., 2008. Modern veterinary graduates are outstanding, but can they get better? J. Vet. Med. Educ. 35 (4), 573–580.

Mylopoulos, M., Regehr, G., 2009. How student models of expertise and innovation impact the development of adaptive expertise in medicine. Med. Educ. 43, 127–132.

Mylopoulos, M., Scardamalia, M., 2008. Doctors' perspectives on their innovations in daily practice: implications for knowledge building in health care. Med. Educ. 42, 975–981.

Oreszczyn, S., Lane, A., Carr, S., 2010. The role of networks of practice and webs of influencers on farmers' engagement with and learning about agricultural innovations. J. Rural Stud. 26, 404–417.

Proctor, A., Lowe, P., Phillipson, J., Donaldson, A., 2011. Veterinary field expertise: using knowledge gained on the job. Vet. Rec. 169, 408–410.

Proctor, A., Donaldson, A., Phillipson, J., Lowe, P., 2012. Field expertise in rural land management. Environment and Planning A 44 (7), 1696–1711.

Rivera, W.M., Sulaiman, V.R., 2009. Extension: object of reform, engine for innovation. Outlook Agr. 38 (3), 267–273.

Swanson, B.E., Bentz, R.P., Sofranko, A.J. (Eds.), 1997. Improving Agricultural Extension: A Reference Manual. FAO, Rome.

Van Crowder, L., Anderson, J., 1997. Linking research, extension and education: why is the problem so persistent and pervasive? Eur. J. Higher Agr. Educ. Ext. 3 (4), 241–250.

PART 2

Practical cases

Ellie Prior: starting out in practice

10

Claire Denny   Sarah Baillie   James Gazzard

CHAPTER OVERVIEW

This fictitious case study is based on Ellie Prior, a typical veterinary graduate taking her first steps into the world of work. While Ellie has been well prepared for the clinical demands she is likely to face, she is less aware and, indeed, less confident of her role as an employee of a small veterinary business. The case aims to explore, through the eyes of a new entrant to the profession, the operations of a typical, small animal veterinary practice. Specifically, it focuses on the challenging topics of talking about money and charging for professional services in a clinical environment.

LEARNING OUTCOMES

After reading this case study, students will be able to:
- Appreciate some of the practical challenges associated with making the transition from 'student' to 'veterinary practitioner'.
- Recognize the form and function of a typical veterinary practice and some of the commercial demands they may face.
- Understand the need to communicate with and take advice from more experienced colleagues within the veterinary practice team.
- Draw on business theories and concepts to suggest what new graduates might do to deal with some of the business challenges presented to Ellie in this case study.

Introduction

Ellie Prior graduated from the Royal Veterinary College, University of London, last summer, aged 23. As she always had a love of animals and a particular interest in animal welfare, her choice to study veterinary medicine was made before she was 10 years old. However, during school she had very little support from teachers. She was told in no uncertain terms by a careers teacher that she might be 'better off lowering her sights to a less competitive and demanding career'. This drove Ellie on to succeed, and her ability to set targets and reach her goals subsequently carried her through five demanding years at the college.

After she bid farewell to her friends at the close of the graduation ceremony, where she was awarded a pass with merit, she drove the two hours home with her proud parents, reflecting on her career ambitions. Her decision had been made some time ago after a pivotal cycle of rotations. Ellie's heart was set on first-opinion small-animal medicine. Making the transition from student to professional was something she had given considerable thought to; being a vet 'for real' is what she had dreamed of and aspired to, but her excitement was tempered with a twinge of doubt. Was she really ready to start out in practice?

Entering the workforce

With her significant student debt weighing heavily on her mind, and her parents' less than subtle reminders of the importance of securing a job, Ellie began to search the veterinary trade press and apply for jobs just one week after the completion of her final exams. After some initial setbacks and useful feedback from a kindly vet during a rejection telephone call, Ellie's luck began to improve.

© 2014, Elsevier Ltd.

Ellie remembered feeling strangely relaxed as she sat on the train flicking through the notes she had prepared for the interview. The interview was surprisingly informal, consisting of a forty-minute chat with the partners, a tour of the facilities and lunch at a local pub with a couple of members of the clinical team. Later that evening she took a deep breath as her phone rang and the practice's number popped up on the display. She had instinctively felt that the practice was an ideal place to commence her career. The call was good news.

Woodall Veterinary Partnership

The busy small-animal practice in which Ellie had secured her first job was located in Woodall, a commuter town of approximately 16 000 people, a ten-minute tram ride from the centre of Birmingham. Having enjoyed life in London while at college, Ellie was keen to move close to another large and vibrant city.

Woodall Vets was a five-vet (including Ellie), four-nurse practice, with one nurse acting as practice manager. There was also a full-time receptionist. It had two branches collectively referred to as the Woodall Veterinary Partnership (WVP). The main branch was in Woodall High Street close to the train station, an off-licence and a growing number of charity shops and estate agents. A smaller satellite branch in Brickall, a small town with approximately 1500 households in a fairly affluent area, helped to widen the caseload. The smaller branch was run by one of the vets, and the nurses rotated to ensure one worked there daily. Routine operations could be performed at Brickall, but any diagnostics and more complicated procedures were sent across to Woodall. WVP had contracted its out-of-hours service to a large nationwide provider of night-time and weekend emergency clinics.

Both sites had been purposely designed, not adapted from existing buildings. The two practices had a light, airy and clean feel to them. A recent improvement project had seen the waiting rooms of both practices redecorated and split into cat- and dog-specific seating areas. Over the years, WVP had developed a strong reputation for delivering high-quality veterinary care.

The practice was founded by Francis Rothwell and Leslie Higgs 34 years ago. Rothwell and Higgs had been friends for almost 40 years, having first met in the student bar when they were undergraduates in Glasgow. They were both straight-talking individuals and excellent vets. They were 'immensely proud' that many of their customers had been loyal to them for 30 years or more. The founding partners had seen the business grow since opening, with the turnover in the last financial year exceeding £750 000 and more than 12 000 patient visits. Julie Butters bought into the practice 5 years ago, having worked for them for 4 years previously. This had allowed the practice to develop with the opening of the Brickall branch, and expansion of the main surgery in Woodall (see Box 10.1).

Both founding partners felt they now wanted more time to enjoy life, having achieved their main professional ambitions. A recent alumni gathering back in Scotland had caused them to think about their futures. A surprising number of their peers had sold their practices to corporate chains and were enjoying the fruits of their retirement. But as Rothwell often put it to their long-standing clients, they 'weren't quite ready to hang up their scalpels'. Instead it was decided that a new vet should be taken on, in the form of Ellie, to allow the older partners to work part-time. Rothwell and Higgs appeared to value the fresh and enthusiastic approach of new graduates, not to mention the lower salary paid to newly qualified members of the profession!

However, Julie, who was still a relatively new partner, was disconcerted that the other partners – who had been energetic and shrewd veterinary entrepreneurs when she first joined the practice almost a decade ago – now seemed happy to take things easy and live off the practice income. Julie's suggestions at the monthly partners' meetings to consider the business case for an extended hours evening surgery one day a week were met with collective dismissive remarks from the founding partners. Her proposal to work with a consultancy that provided feedback on the practice through mystery shoppers was quietly ignored. After long tiring days, Julie often commented to her husband that she was doing 'far more than her fair share'. She craved a better work–life balance. Julie was also growing increasingly frustrated with Rothwell and Higgs' almost daily trips to the off-licence to buy a 'nice Rioja' to accompany their early and extended lunch breaks where they chatted about 'the good old days' in the upstairs office. She had begun to think about starting a family in the near future before it was 'too late', but could not see how this would fit in with the clinical and commercial demands of the practice.

Having previously had limited competition from neighbouring practices, WVP had developed a healthy income stream. However, the national chain 'Pet SuperSaver' had recently applied to the local council

Box 10.1

SWOT analysis for Woodall Veterinary Partnership (prepared by Julie Butters during an external practice management workshop)

Strengths	Weaknesses	Opportunities	Threats
• Woodhall: central location in middle-class town • Brickall: only practice in affluent town • Strong clinical team • Solid client base, growing business • Ample parking at both practices • Reputation for high-quality veterinary care and compassionate nurses • Practice owns land/building, no rent	• No marketing (apart from occasional small advert in parish magazine) • No website. No Facebook site • Restricted opening hours • Brickall branch: limited diagnostic equipment and surgical space • Limited training provided to reception staff	• Starting to use new 360-degree performance review to improve service • Could use the new 'What's on in Woodall' community website for marketing • To increase satellite branch turnover/size • To get more involved in community events (something that had been turned down due to lack of time before) • Open evenings, puppy parties	• Founding partners now want to spend more time away from practice, soon to retire and will need buying out • Loyal customers may leave practice when partners retire • Current Internet drug companies providing cheaper drugs • Large, low-cost, pet superstore (with vet practice) due to open shortly

for planning permission to open a large outlet on a retail estate less than a 5-minute drive from Woodall. The planning application stated that a veterinary practice franchise would be included in the store. The new store would certainly encroach on WVP's catchment area. Ellie had worked in a Pet SuperSaver practice two summers ago during a hastily arranged fortnight of extramural study. She recalled early-morning meetings with the area manager who reviewed the branch's performance. There was much talk of 'performance metrics': number of appointments and follow-ups booked, average consult times, target transaction value for each vet as well as price benchmarks against local practices, percentage of clients buying flea treatments and wormers. One vet she shadowed was keen to tell her that his sporty new car was bought with last year's performance bonus. The workplace culture of the Pet SuperSaver practice was something Ellie had not experienced before. She had mixed feelings. The clients certainly seemed to value the competitively priced service, Sunday opening and ample free parking. However, she felt a little uneasy and surprised when the vets spent an afternoon on sales training. Ellie wondered what effect the new store would have on her future at WVP. Julie and Ellie had already overheard some of their customers enthusiastically talking about the possibility of getting vaccinations at the new store for 'less than half the price' charged by the WVP practices.

Ellie felt the Woodall practice was a good fit for her first job; she was grateful for the support of Julie, who gave her plenty of responsibility, and allowed her to follow through her own cases and make her own decisions. Julie was always available for friendly guidance and a helping hand, although Ellie was concerned that she was a drain on Julie's time. Julie had told Ellie she had the potential to be a great vet, but had a lot to learn. The nurses had generally made her transition much smoother, often giving Ellie the impression they were coaxing her in the right direction! Last week a couple of regular clients had even specifically asked to see 'that nice new vet, Ellie', which gave a boost to her confidence.

Six months on

On a dark and cold February early evening Ellie sat with a steaming hot cup of tea at the rear of the practice in an untidy space that doubled as the staff room and cleaning cupboard. Her 6-month review, which had taken place earlier in the day, had been a useful experience. The partners had collected feedback on her performance from the clinical team, the receptionists and a small selection of clients. Julie had called it a 360-degree review process, and had seemed more excited by the new way of conducting performance reviews than the older partners. Ellie had been relieved that all parties were satisfied with her clinical skills – although Rothwell had muttered something about her needing to speed up her consults. However, Higgs gave her some feedback from George, the vet who normally worked at the Brickall practice, that her diagnostic and client-facing skills were 'coming along nicely'. Julie had mentioned the prospect of Ellie attending a 2-day course in canine oncology as a number of dogs being treated by the practice were undergoing chemotherapy. All things considered, Ellie was delighted with the comments; she had loved her first 6 months at WVP.

Then, towards the end of the meeting, Rothwell began to talk about a recent drive her boss had taken across to the retail park where the Pet SuperSaver store was under construction. Ellie too had seen the cavernous steel superstructure when she had been out shopping the previous Sunday. Rothwell struggled to hide his concern. While he made some comments about how confident they were that WVP's 'exemplary' level of customer service would continue to help their business to thrive, it was noted in an ominous tone that they would need to 'up their game'. Ellie had overheard Rothwell and Higgs recently making comments about the new generation of vets 'living in cloud cuckoo land' about the realities of running a successful small, independent, veterinary business. Ellie guessed what was

coming next. Julie started to talk about a couple of incidents that had happened in close succession a couple of weeks before Christmas. At the time Higgs had summoned Ellie into the upstairs office and called them 'beginners' mistakes' and began to give her a well-meaning but grumpy lecture on 'cash flow'; she remembered the partner repeating, at least three times, that 'money in the till is the lifeblood of any small business'. Julie said that she had seen this time and time again – early-career vets overlooking the importance of charging appropriately for their time. The partners concluded by asking Ellie to really give this matter some thought, stating that they would be keeping a careful eye on her progress.

As Ellie sipped her tea she started to reflect on the two incidents the partners had spoken about. What had caused them? Were there particular patterns in her behaviour that had triggered the events? Were there critical gaps in her knowledge and skills? Had she spent enough time learning about the practice as a business and considering her role within it? Would being 'too business minded' as a vet compromise her role as a clinician? What could she do to respond to the partners' feedback? Determined to become a well-rounded practitioner she played the two incidents over in her mind. On her smartphone she used a free app she had found to help her to capture her initial thoughts (see Box 10.2).

Box 10.2

Performance appraisal framework from a smart phone app (recorded by Ellie Prior)

Excellence	Accountability	Teamwork	Customer service	Integrity	Professional development
• Is clinical excellence enough? • Should I be contributing more to the business at this stage of my career? If so, what? • Perhaps I want to own a practice in the future – not sure. What would it take to be a successful veterinary entrepreneur?	• I don't know how much I am earning for the practice • Do I earn more than I cost the practice in salary, National Insurance, pension and other costs? • Am I confident enough to charge what I am worth? • I am not really sure what the business wants from me	• Could we do more collectively as a team to improve the business? Team targets? • I don't speak with the partners and other members of the team enough about the commercial aspects of practice	• Clients ask me to do the best I can for the animal and then complain when they pay the bill • How do I talk to clients about money? • Am I an advocate for clients or the practice?	• I am not a sales person • I am on the side of the client and their pets • It's not all about money • But on the other hand, I expect my salary to be paid each month	• What do I need to do to improve my business awareness? • Could I find a mentor to help me learn more about the business aspects of practice? • Perhaps a business night class at the local FE college?

Incident 1: the easier way out of a difficult situation

Rory, a 3-year-old male Springer Spaniel, gashed his right forelimb while out walking on Woodall Heath with his owner Natalie Parr. His concerned owner took him straight to the practice and asked if Rory could be seen by a vet as soon as possible.

Ellie was feeling the strain of a long morning which had been fully booked-up with 10-minute consults, and a receptionist who insisted on remarking to every customer at the desk 'It's the new young vet this morning. She's very good, but a bit slow.' Ellie gave up what was left of her lunch break to see the extremely excitable, tail-wagging, Rory.

Usually Ellie enjoyed the bouncy nature of Springers, but today she just wanted 10 minutes to put her aching feet up and rest. She promptly took a look at the dog's leg, finding a 6 cm simple wound. Since it was fresh, Ellie decided to debride and suture the wound, finally applying a bandage, pleased that she did not need to spend too much time in the small consulting room. On handing Rory back to his owner, Ellie informed Miss Parr that she would need to bring the dog back to the practice to be re-examined in 5 days, or sooner if there was any sign of discharge or the bandage got wet. The client paid and seemed pleased that her beloved Rory had suffered no lasting damage.

As requested, Rory returned in 5 days. Ellie checked with Miss Parr if there had been any problems with Rory, and heard that he had been getting on absolutely fine. Miss Parr was then told that her dog would be taken to the hospital area in order for the wound to be checked and the bandage reapplied, and that perhaps she could pay her bill (see Box 10.3) at the reception while she waited. The owner seemed confused, believing that the re-examination cost was included in last week's 'not inconsiderable' bill. She

enquired forcefully whether she really had to pay as all Ellie was going to do was change a bandage, which 'she could have done herself'.

Ellie, feeling quite agitated by this remark, told the client that she was paying for a medical professional's time to view a wound, and that 'any professional, whether it be a plumber or a lawyer' would expect to be compensated for the time they spent with clients. Bluntly, Miss Parr launched into a monologue debasing the position of vets, saying how those in a caring profession 'overcharged caring pet owners', just as she 'had seen on an undercover television programme last month'. Ellie, thinking about the long list of clients facing her later that afternoon, told Miss Parr that the fee would be waived.

Ellie did not give the matter much further thought until she was called to Higgs' office. The partner had not long come off the phone from Miss Parr, and was now late for his lunch meeting with the practice's accountant. Higgs was very disappointed that now they had 'the worst of both worlds': an unhappy client and no income from the consult.

Incident 2: sensitive issues around fees and billing

Ellie found herself alone in the practice. Both founding partners had left before midday in readiness for an afternoon at Brickall Golf and Country Club, and Julie had booked the afternoon off. All parties were more than confident that Ellie could cope with the appointments, which consisted mainly of routine vaccinations and re-exams. If help was required, George, a more experienced vet at the Brickall practice, was available.

After finishing off the morning's work, phoning clients with results and typing up her notes, Ellie was warned by the receptionist that a dog involved in a road traffic accident was being brought in to be treated; sadly, from the garbled message it sounded unlikely that the dog would survive. Ellie quickly telephoned George. After what felt like an age on hold, but was probably only a couple of minutes, George picked up the phone and explained he had a waiting room full of patients and was 'flat out'. Ellie explained the situation and George offered a few words of reassurance, mentioned something about the practice's 'PTS (put to sleep) policy' and wished her good luck. Ellie's mind was racing.

Box 10.3

Rory (Miss Parr) re-examination bill
Invoice: Woodall Veterinary Partnership

Breakdown	Price
Re-examine fee	£25.73
Small bandage	£15.52
Sub-total	£41.25
VAT	£8.25
Total	£49.50

IMMEDIATE PAYMENT DUE

A few minutes later the dog arrived. Ellie promptly examined the West Highland White Terrier. She instantly realized that the dog was suffering greatly and urgently needed to be euthanized. Ellie looked up and remembered that she had not acknowledged the elderly couple in front of her. A white-haired man, who Ellie guessed was in his eighties, stood quietly. A smartly dressed lady, of a similar age, who Ellie presumed to be his wife, was speaking quickly and in tears. The woman snapped at the man: 'You should never have been driving, with your eyesight.' The woman pleaded with Ellie to do whatever she could to help the dog.

Ellie communicated calmly and precisely that the dog was severely injured and was in a state of extreme pain and the proper medical decision, indeed the right ethical choice, would be to stop this animal's suffering. The elderly man finally spoke, seemingly riddled with guilt, and begged Ellie to try to save the dog. He then added: 'Are you sure you know what you are doing? You look younger than my granddaughter.' Ellie, with an air of authority which belied her nerves, told the couple that the animal needed to be 'put to sleep'. After a brief discussion, the couple reluctantly agreed. The lady immediately became reserved and silent after signing the consent form. Ellie swiftly prepared and conducted the procedure; talking to the animal softly through its final moments. Shortly afterwards the couple then began to make their way out of the practice.

Ellie felt the adrenalin leave her body as she and Jody, a nurse, cleaned the consult room. Jody asked how things had gone. Ellie replayed the incident out loud to Jody. Immediately Ellie realized her mistake. The couple had left and not paid for the procedure or the disposal of the animal. Ellie suddenly recalled the PTS policy George had mentioned on the phone, and which she knew well already. A check of the reception team found that they had not seen the couple previously, had no contact details for them and were listed only as Mr and Mrs Jones. The corner of Ellie's eye flicked across to a clear sign behind the reception desk that stated the practice's policy of 'no accounts', 'no credit' and 'immediate payment'.

Looking back on the two incidents, Ellie wondered how she might have handled things differently. As she finished her tea, she started to think about some business management books she had read recently; perhaps she could use some of the ideas she had picked up in those to ensure she did not make the same mistakes again?

Declaration

The authors declare that the characters, veterinary-sector businesses and geographical settings depicted in this case study are fictitious, and any similarities to real people (living or deceased), trading or defunct veterinary-sector businesses or places are unintentional.

Acknowledgements

The authors would like to thank the veterinary practitioners who gave their time to respond to surveys and face-to-face interviews in order to inform the content of this fictitious case study.

Church Hill Equine Clinic: changing large-animal practice in rural areas

11

Izzy Warren Smith

CASE OVERVIEW

This case study maps the successful start-up, survival and growth of a large-animal veterinary practice located in the Welsh–English borderlands. It identifies the key factors that have precipitated and facilitated growth, and traces the progression of the business from a rural large-animal practice to a specialist equine clinic. Issues such as practice specialization, profitability, marketing, staffing and the changing rural market for veterinary practice are addressed. The case provides students with a 'real-life' scenario to which they can apply business and enterprise theory, and from which they can learn about the practicalities of running a rural-based veterinary enterprise.

LEARNING OUTCOMES

After reading this case study, students will be able to:
- Understand the difficulties associated with running a rural veterinary practice.
- Appreciate some of the complexities associated with growing a veterinary practice in a rural location.
- Draw on business and enterprise theory to explore some of the potential strategies available to Church Hill and propose a future direction for the business.

Introduction

The financial end-of-year partners' meeting of Church Hill Equine Clinic ended with an agreement to review the business's strategic direction. The partners had discussed trying to further expand the regional market share of the practice over the next year. In short, the business was reasonably successful but not operating optimally. Things had to change, but with a six-vet practice operating from three separate home locations, and a business built on the reputation and charisma of its two founding partners, it was not going to be easy. However, the announcement at the same meeting that Rhys, one of the senior founding partners wanted to go part-time and eventually retire caused Rob Pitt, the most recent senior partner, to start thinking about how he might grow the business into the future.

Background

Prior to joining Church Hill, Rob Pitt had spent some time in a large-animal mixed practice in the northwest of England. This involved miscellaneous practice experience across mainly cattle and horses. However, after 3 years he realized that his daily work had become mundane and routine. It was clear to him that any concentration on bovines would mean his work was focused around herd health planning and production management, with little or no contact with individual animals. It was also clear that economics dictated the owner's decisions, and in the event of anything being found wrong with an animal, it was a simple matter of 'shoot and replace'.

As a vet, Rob had always been more interested in working with and treating the individual animal, and realized that with equine his job was more varied, challenging and professionally stretching. Rob had enjoyed the equine part more and more, eventually splitting his time between equine and bovine work. He had a farming background, and was increasingly conscious that when equine customers called the

© 2014, Elsevier Ltd.

large-animal mixed practice they always wanted 'the horse vet'. The other vets in the practice preferred to leave the equine work to him and, as a consequence, he received an increasing number of referrals within the practice. All this experience, Rob realized, had stood him in good stead prior to joining Church Hill.

As Rob reflected on the past 12 years of his part-nership at the practice, he remembered that when he originally joined there was a period of recession. The practice had been started by Rhys Evans as a large-animal practice. Rhys was a high-profile and locally well-known popular vet who had returned 'home' to rural Wales, having spent some time working over-seas and then at the Royal College of Veterinary Surgeons (RCVS) doing surgery. During this time he had developed an interest in equine medicine, but he continued with large-animal practice as the dictates of the local rural economy demanded. A year later, he was joined by Daffyd, who was an equine enthusiast, a well-known character within the local equine community, and keen on hunting and 'point to point'. Both Rhys and Daffyd were self-employed and worked from their separate home bases, but decided that they would operate under the banner of Church Hill Equine Vets. As such they formed a two-location practice, Rhys in Llanyfirs and Daffyd just over the English border, close to a county town. Their respective reputations along with their client base grew steadily. Five years from inception, and under their charismatic leadership, they additionally took on another vet partner and, 3 years after that, Rob Pitt. As the number of vets grew, the business continued to grow exponentially, despite the reces-sion; the practice supply of high-quality equine vets remained unable to outstrip demand for them.

Church Hill Equine Clinic was becoming more established, albeit still a 'loose association' of self-employed vets operating from two senior partner home bases. This was primarily driven by a combination of the character and reputation and, by extension, the individ-ual 'brands' of Rhys and Daffyd, respectively. They had never felt the need to advertise, having operated at a time when competition was virtually non-existent. Most large-animal vets were mixed practice, and equine vets were still something of a novelty.

From fast start to plateau

The number of partners in the practice had increased in the 12 years since Rob had started. Six vets (one of whom was an associate partner) were now operating

under the banner of Church Hill, although founder partner Rhys had recently indicated his desire to go part-time and eventually retire. There had also been a number of very discernible changes. In the early days, there had not been many horse-specialist veterinary practices around. Cattle and large-animal mixed-practice vets were disinclined to treat horses, so Church Hill would get plenty of 'business-to-business' referrals from other practices. However, Rob had begun to notice that, as time went on, more and more practices wanted to get involved in equine work, and as a consequence the number of equine vets had increased. This trend could be directly related to the farming recession, which saw dairy farmers go out of production while equine businesses were still a growing rural industry. Needless to say, Rob had started to see an increase in competition. In the past, he had sug-gested taking a half-page advertisement in Yellow Pages, much to the resistance of the older senior part-ners, who failed to see the need at that time. His obser-vation now was that Church Hill, with the growth in the number of vets operating from the practice, would soon need to do much more marketing. However, by this stage, things had moved well beyond just placing an advertisement in Yellow Pages.

With Rob becoming a senior partner, practice pre-mises still consisted of 'home-based' clinics, but based at the homes of the now three senior partners (Rhys, Daffyd and Rob), which were located in rural Wales, the outskirts of a border English county town and a village in rural England. These three locations were serviced by the other self-employed partners and associate, who paid surgery rental to the respec-tive location partners. Rhys's retirement would mean the loss of one of these surgery bases.

Although the practice was continuing to grow, the client base had started to plateau as local compe-tition increased. Similarly, Rob had noticed a slight change in the demographics of the practice customer base, with more of the clients now coming from England. With the main surgical base still in Llanyfir (Rhys's home), this was causing logistical difficulties. Partnership vets were contributing to surgery rental dependent on where they saw clients and which rota was in operation, but rentals were not charged at com-mercial rates due to the home-based nature of the business.

To date, all capital investment was in skills, drugs and equipment rather than in property. The process of travelling was becoming increasingly awkward and, as expertise and clinical provision became more spe-cialized, the need for higher-specification equipment increased. The two portable X-ray machines were not always efficient. They took time to process and read, resulting in considerable delays between X-ray, customer feedback and animal treatment. Similarly, providing more advanced veterinary treatment was curtailed by the fragmented locations. Rob began to see both the opportunity and the need for significant and fundamental changes.

Going for growth

Rob decided to develop his small surgery by investing in a purpose-built clinic at his home, located in an English border village, which was in between the original previous two locations. This was largely in response to client geography and demand. The fully equipped clinic had a dramatic effect on the practice, and there was a subsequent 'explosion' of business growth. Prior to the new clinic, the practice's English-based clients had never had a permanent location as a focal point for the practice – a location that they could recognize as a fully equipped clinic. The practice quickly grew from six to ten vets, along with support staff, to keep up with increased demand and output, totalling 16 staff in all. The new developments, which had really revolutionized Church Hill, were working far better for both client and veterinarian alike. The practice was still 'Church Hill' but facilities were better, with, for example, one very high-specification 'fixed' X-ray machine, rather than two smaller, less efficient mobile X-ray units. It was better to have one good-quality machine in a single location and benefit from higher output.

It became easier to take X-rays, and both efficiency and output increased as more horses came in for lameness work-ups and assessments. The equipment was able to produce better-quality images that could be diagnosed quickly while the client was still on site, and client satisfaction increased. Similarly, throughput had increased as a result of the development of new operating theatres and assessment rooms. The practice could now undertake complex colic and orthopaedic surgeries without having to keep disassembling and reassembling all the complex surgical equipment. The inclusion of a knock-down box, pulley, gantry and a scrubbing-up room for preparation, along with other new facilities, meant that the practice could have several procedures going on at the same time. The new comprehensive facilities now included:

- padded induction ('drop boxes') boxes for anaesthesia;
- space for remedial farriery;
- new operating theatre (see Figure 11.1);
- scrub-up room;
- examination room;
- stock and store room;
- office room;
- reception area;
- paddock space and lameness work-up areas.
- on-site practice laboratory

Rob Pitt's personal capital investment had essentially resourced Church Hill's infrastructural and business growth. To start with, out of respect for the way the practice had originally operated, Rob only charged rental for the administrative office, as the two founder partners still had 'practice stables' and clinics at their homes. Rob felt that the move had sufficiently benefited him as a partner, given that the new facilities were on his home site. He was not too bothered about

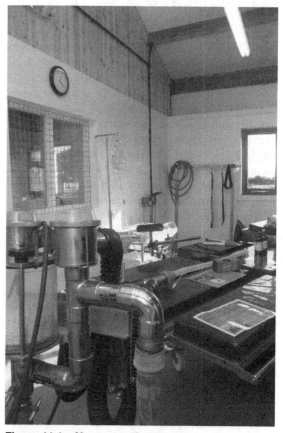

Figure 11.1 • New operating theatre

rent in the short term, as he considered that the expansion was a reasonable investment in the long term. Rob continued the site expansion and development of the practice's clinical facilities. He had sufficient space and maintained a constant vision for opportunity exploitation, progress and business growth, all under the banner of a higher-quality service and improved provision for customers.

Human resourcing and growing pains

As with any business development where there has been significant expansion, human resources had to be developed to facilitate growth. When recruiting, Church Hill had originally targeted veterinary staff with specialist equine skills. However, experience showed them that while candidates often had impressive equine experience on paper, this did not always work well in practice once candidates were hired. When they got into the routine of Church Hill's rural location, new staff often did not 'fit' with the practice's caseload. In some cases individual staff members were so specialist that 'they weren't able to cope with the routine mundane work that sometimes needed to be done, like vaccines, fetal scanning, etc.' Church Hill quickly realized that there was a difference between the work the candidates thought they would be doing and what they actually did. In reality there are not many practices that can 'just do surgery' all day outside of a university location, except in the south of England or by the racecourses. Eventually, Church Hill recognized that what it actually needed was staff who were essentially generalists but had an equine focus.

The practice decided to adopt a policy of taking recent veterinary graduates who could be trained in the 'Church Hill mind set' and educated about its value system along the way. This resulted in better experience all round and created a better working environment. The practice was big enough for graduates to learn and benefit from a range of expertise. This way, Church Hill was able to train the graduates to fit the practice's culture, noting that 'the habits you build up are the habits you want to build up'. All of this is driven by their understanding that 'the customer's perception is very important'. As Rob observed:

> From the client's perspective, if a graduate comes to Church Hill, they are immediately a 'horse vet', as they

are operating under the Church Hill banner, whereas in mixed practice it's hard to specialize even if you are interested. In large mixed practice everyone wants 'the horse vet' and in a mixed practice you're never likely going to be 'the horse vet' when you first start.

The supply of veterinary graduates in the last 4–5 years has changed dramatically. Not only has there been an increase in the number of vets, but there are also more graduates wanting to undertake equine vet practice. Five years ago, most of the partners and associates who applied to Church Hill were male; now most of the applications are from female veterinarians, and the female vets who have joined the team thus far have chosen to remain as associates rather than partners.

Support staff

The support office staff team has also expanded in line with the growth of Church Hill. Indeed, when the new purpose-built premises were being developed, they appointed a new practice/office manager. New systems were set up, and the office and administrative side of things were working more smoothly as a result. However, there were problems with the wider office team who objected to being line managed by an 'office manager'; essentially, they wanted the vets to be in charge.

The original practice manager subsequently left and another manager was recruited; however, it was eventually decided to divide the administrative roles amongst the remaining office staff. Each office team member was given specific responsibility for one of the office outputs. For example, one staff member who was particularly successful with client debt management was given control of that function. The office staff members now work as a real team; this system seems to work well. The net result has been a clear delineation, with veterinary partners as 'managers' and administrative staff as 'service providers' supporting the overall 'Church Hill team' effort. Regular practice meetings were now taking place with a collaborative approach to new ideas and development.

Marketing

Church Hill was, once again, facing increasing competition. Graduates have come out of vet schools and started equine practices. In the past it was not a popular target market for large-animal practice.

As such, Church Hill, having plateaued at the ten-vet stage, has to work harder to keep its clients. The partners now have to reinforce relationships to maintain their dominance of the local equine market, as Rob observed:

> Word of mouth and reputation was always sufficient in the past, which, although even now is still the best form of marketing, is no longer enough.

As such more advertising and marketing have become necessary.

Their competitors have adopted an aggressive marketing strategy, including going from [other practice customer's equine] yard to yard and producing advertising leaflets. This has upset other local practices, but the new vets seem untroubled by this. As Rob noted:

> New graduates are coming out with a very different philosophy and this would never have happened before.

Business strategy

Rob is now principal partner and is keen to keep moving the practice forward; he wants to retain the good staff he has recruited and continue providing a high-quality service. Conscious that the business is for the customers and that without them he has no business, he needs to think carefully about the way forward. He knows too that customers may not be fully aware of just how much his team can provide with the practice's newly equipped and functioning facilities.

As a practice, partners no longer cover the huge distances they once did, and are increasingly finding that people are travelling to them. There is definitely more competition on the periphery of their boundaries but, despite this, there is still a growing number of horses coming into the surgery for treatment. Rob is concerned about this and wonders if this boundary retraction, while still maintaining the client base and output, is a result of an increase in the number of horses locally, or due to other factors.

A range of opportunities and options are open to the practice, and these will involve a number of collaborative relationships. Such relationships need to be cultivated in order to develop the service provision for clients so that they use Church Hill in preference to other competitors. Rob has, for example, recently managed to set up a preferential partnership arrangement with a pharmaceutical company to develop further business.

Vet practices now struggle to compete on price with businesses such as farmer suppliers and country stores. One example of this is the provision of wormers; essentially, the practice was missing an 'add-on' sales opportunity. To counter this, Church Hill has started providing a worm egg count service using its on-site labs. Worming, as a service, targets worm populations, replacing worming rotations with egg counts and targeted treatment, which is generally now recognized to be better practice. Rob has combined this with sales of targeted wormers, once specific parasites have been identified. The new lab facilities are now being used more efficiently and, by providing a paid-for service, have become cost effective.

Moving forward: developing a vision for the future

Rob feels that Church Hill still has considerable growth potential. However, he feels that the practice site is already operating at optimum size with 16 staff. This comprises ten vets, six of whom are now partners, with four associates and six office staff to support the practice. He wants to maintain a leading equine practice and continue to provide a high-quality service. While there are probably several different growth models that he could adopt, for the moment 'there is no mission, no clear vision as such; it's more a case of just keeping things ticking along nicely'.

Church Hill has certainly come a long way from the charismatic branding that revolved around its two founding partners. Staff meetings, for example, are much more positive now, with lots of new ideas brought forward and the younger partners' fresh thinking keeping everyone keener and sharper. Whereas in the past Rob struggled to get his colleagues' support for basic marketing activities, now there is a sense of positive collaboration and enthusiasm for driving the business forward.

Much of Church Hill's future now lies with the practice's forward-thinking young veterinary team and the new graduates that will be recruited as the practice continues to grow. Rob is mindful of changes in the veterinary market place, increasing competition and the need to maintain a high-quality service. While he is confident that Church Hill has the potential to maintain its market lead, he remains undecided as to which particular business strategy he will need to adopt to make this happen.

12

Cromlyn Vets: where to now?

Colette Henry

CHAPTER OVERVIEW

This case study focuses on a small mixed veterinary practice in Northern Ireland, established by husband and wife team Chris and Lynn Heffron. The growth and development of the business are discussed, along with the various challenges the business has had to face in its near 30-year history. The case focuses on practical veterinary business issues such as striving for and maintaining excellence in clinical veterinary care, maximizing resources, utilizing available expertise and retaining client numbers in the face of growing competition.

LEARNING OUTCOMES

After reading this case study, students will be able to:
- Understand the challenges involved in developing and growing a small veterinary practice.
- Appreciate the need to develop a strategic marketing plan to deal with growing competition.
- Apply marketing theories to propose a strategy for addressing the challenge now facing Cromlyn Vets and determine the way forward.

Introduction

When you first walk into Cromlyn House Veterinary Hospital you are immediately struck by its sheer brightness, freshness and cleanliness. Despite its rural location, it has the look and feel of an urban facility, with the latest in surgical equipment, balanced with a spacious and welcoming reception area. Cromlyn's in-house laboratory enables rapid and accurate analysis of blood, urine and cytology samples, while

sophisticated X-ray, ultrasound and endoscopy equipment allow for immediate on-site patient diagnosis. Of course, all of this is hardly surprising, given that Cromlyn Vets is one of only two RCVS (Royal College of Veterinary Surgeons) accredited Tier 3 small-animal hospitals in Northern Ireland (NI). However, achieving and maintaining such high standards of excellence in veterinary care take hard work, dedication and a highly qualified team of professionals – essential components of any successful business. In developing Cromlyn from a small husband-and-wife start-up practice into a professional state-of-the-art veterinary hospital, with an annual turnover in excess of £1 million, principal partners Chris and Lynn Heffron have had a lot of tough decisions to make along the way. Reflecting on their *veterinary business journey* so far, and mindful of rumours of imminent corporate entry into the NI marketplace, they suddenly realize that they have even more important decisions to make if they are to secure the future of the successful business they have spent nearly 30 years developing.

Background

Cromlyn House Veterinary Hospital was established in 1985 by Chris and Lynn Heffron as a small-animal/ equine veterinary practice. Based in Hillsborough, Northern Ireland, the business started out as a 'partnership' but is now a limited company with a total of 16 staff. When it first opened its doors to the public, the practice was based in an old terraced building in the main street of the village of Hillsborough (Figure 12.1). While its original client base comprised

© 2014, Elsevier Ltd.

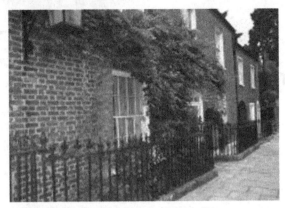

Figure 12.1 • Cromlyn Vets' original site
Source: www.cromlynvets.ac.uk

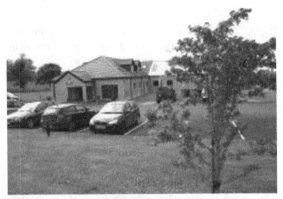

Figure 12.2 • Cromlyn Vets' current premises
Source: www.cromlynvets.ac.uk

50% equine and 50% small animal, as the practice expanded it became clear that this dual service was going to be increasingly difficult to maintain. Thus Chris and Lynn made the difficult decision to focus entirely on small-animal practice and, as a result, moved out of the centre of the village to a new location that they felt would be more convenient for their clients. In 2002, a new purpose-built Cromlyn Veterinary Hospital was opened exactly one mile from the site of the original practice (Figure 12.2). The practice's immediate geographical area is Hillsborough, County Down, and greater Belfast; however, the practice's client base actually spans the whole of Northern Ireland, often taking referrals from as far away as Derry and the northwest.

The Cromlyn veterinary team

In addition to Chris and Lynn, the Cromlyn team comprises experienced and dedicated vets, veterinary nurses, receptionists and cleaning staff, who

collectively enable the practice to provide specialized services in small-animal surgery, ophthalmology and orthopaedics. A specialist vet cardiologist and orthopaedic surgeon also attend the Cromlyn practice to carry out more sophisticated procedures when required. In addition, the practice provides a wide range of pet care services, including health checks, inoculation, neutering (dogs and cats), dental hygiene and blood tests; and boasts a suite of dedicated surgical and dental theatres, as well as dog and cat wards with round-the-clock nursing care. Services are also provided for new puppies and kittens as well as ageing pets, and specialist advice on breeding and diet is also available. More recent services include microchipping, pet passports and pet cremation. Locally, the practice works closely with a number of NI-based animal charities and rehoming organizations, and treats local wildlife casualties free of charge.

Chris Heffron, the managing partner, qualified as a veterinary surgeon from Glasgow University in 1973, and subsequently spent a few years in practice in both NI and South Africa. He also lectured in Glasgow in surgical anatomy. He then moved to the Curragh in Kildare, where he worked mainly with racehorses. He holds a Masters degree (MVM) in ENT surgery. While Chris was always keen to have his own veterinary business, on reflection he admits that:

Starting a business from scratch was probably not the right way to do things – it was very challenging, particularly financially. I probably should have joined a large partnership first and then worked my way up to partner level; the way I did it really was a lot of hard work!

Prior to setting up Cromlyn Vets with Chris, Lynn spent some time working in mixed practice in NI before taking up a post at the SPCA (Society for the Prevention of Cruelty to Animals) in Cape Town. She then returned to Glasgow, her alma mater, to complete a Masters degree in orthopaedics.

The 'business' of veterinary medicine!

Chris and Lynn both believe that business skills are hugely important for veterinarians, but reflecting on their undergraduate years they both recall that there were no business or enterprise skills provided in their veterinary curriculum, as Chris explains:

We got no training at all, which is probably why we weren't very good at managing the business side of things in the beginning, and we certainly weren't prepared for the many business challenges we faced.

More specifically, Chris identifies computing skills as being critical to running a veterinary practice, as clinical records, client and supplier databases and pricing systems are all IT-based. He is aware that more benefit could be derived for the practice if they were able to fully exploit their computer systems, i.e. avail themselves of detailed reporting functions and client analysis. With regard to the latter, Chris clearly places considerable importance on customer relations, striving to ensure that:

We treat every client as a new client and update our records every time the customer visits; this gives us a chance to further engage with them too; good interpersonal skills are really important, especially if you are trying to build up a new practice. Practices grow by word of mouth; clients have to leave your practice feeling good, so good consulting and communication skills are critical.

Thus consultation, general practice management and marketing are all critical skills required to successfully set up and manage a veterinary practice. According to Chris, it is important to include these sorts of business and management skills in the undergraduate veterinary curriculum because, while CPD (continuous professional development) courses are great, when you are a practising vet your time becomes very limited and such courses can be quite expensive.

Managing the money

Good cash-flow management is critical to any business, but it can be a particular issue in veterinary practice. Cash flow is all about 'getting the money in' and charging in an appropriate and timely manner; this means being 'upfront' when you are talking to your clients about pricing. As Chris explains:

Interestingly, some people can get quite embarrassed when they have to talk about money. People typically go into veterinary practice as a career because they want to do good, which is great, but veterinary practice is essentially 'private practice' and we need to be able to talk about money without feeling embarrassed. You really need to be talking to your clients all the time about the money side of things, not leaving it till the

end and then just produce a big bill – that can be really unfair on your client.

Chris admits that money is not such an issue with insured pets, but only 20% of Cromlyn clients actually have pet insurance, a figure the practice is keen to increase in the coming years. The key thing to remember is that 'you could lose a client on the basis of your failure to talk about money rather than on the basis of poor veterinary work', hence the need to be 'upfront' with your client about the cost of the veterinary care you are recommending.

The veterinary marketplace

In 2012, the UK dog population was estimated at around 8 million. During the same year, the UK cat population was also estimated at around 8 million (PFMA, 2012). Table 12.1 shows a breakdown of other different pets in the UK.

In Ireland, 2006 statistics revealed that there were an estimated 640 000 pet dog-owning, and 215 542 pet cat-owning households. Overall, almost one in two households (i.e. 22 million households) in the UK owned a pet in 2011. Based on this ratio, it is estimated that 388 000 households in NI keep a pet (Downes et al., 2011).

In terms of veterinary employment, according to Lantra (2011), of the 47 500 people employed in veterinary activities in the UK, around 500 (about 1%) are employed in NI across the province's 140 or so veterinary businesses. Such statistics are important when trying to develop an effective and appropriate marketing strategy for the business. In this regard, part of Cromlyn's core marketing strategy includes maintaining their comprehensive website and providing a monthly client newsletter with updates, free pet care advice and promotional offers. Client queries can also be addressed via the website, and appointments can be made online. The practice also runs open evenings, puppy parties and open days for existing and prospective clients. In addition, a 'question and answer' session is provided for the general public via a weekly column in a local newspaper.

More recently, Cromlyn launched its new online veterinary store, where clients can browse through a range of pet foods and nutritional supplements from leading suppliers, make their purchase and collect their goods at a pre-arranged time. Cromlyn will typically text their clients to let them know when their goods are ready for collection.

Table 12.1 UK pet population breakdown in 2012

Dogs	8 million (approx. 23% of UK households have at least one dog)
Cats	8 million (approx. 19% of UK households have at least one cat)
Indoor fish	20–25 million kept in tanks
Outdoor Fish	20–25 million kept in ponds
Rabbits	1 million
Caged birds	1 million
Guinea-pigs	1 million
Hamsters	500 000
Domestic fowl	500 000
Horses/ponies	100 000
Tortoises/turtles	200 000
Gerbils	100 000
Snakes	200 000
Lizards	300 000
Rats	200 000
Frogs and toads	200 000
Newts/salamanders	100 000
Mice	Fewer than 100 000 people keep mice
Insects	Fewer than 100 000 people keep insects

Source: Pet Food Manufacturers' Association, available from http://www.pfma.org.uk/pet-population/

The changing veterinary business landscape

Chris, Lynn and the team are mindful of the many changes taking place in the veterinary business landscape. For example, there has been some evidence of unemployment within the sector, perhaps a reflection of the current recession. In this regard, he cites an example of how Cromlyn Vets recently advertised for a 6-month maternity replacement and were inundated with inquiries:

> There are a lot of vet graduates now – it may be that there are too many for all of them to get full employment?

However, the salaries of vets are nowhere near those of GPs, despite the tough competition for places in veterinary medicine and the high academic entry requirements. A young GP I know had initially been interested in becoming a vet but told me that she didn't get the grades for vet school so ended up taking medicine instead!

The current recession also means that there is a general downturn in elective spending by the population, and this affects everyone. According to Chris, 'people are tightening their belts when it comes to discretionary spending'.

The rapid feminization of the profession has also had an impact on the sector, with the overwhelming majority of veterinary graduates now being female. He believes that this may have implications for farm animal practices, as he explains:

> Some women choose to go into farm animal practice and do very well, but farm practices are contracting. However, there shouldn't be a problem for equine – lots of women do really well in this sector due to early childhood equine interests and activities. Actually, the arrival of the 'married part-time female vet' is a very positive thing for the profession; it means that there are lots of locums available to practices, and part-time flexible work options available to vets when needed.

Moving forward: competing with the corporates

The threat of corporate entry into the NI veterinary sector, something not seen as a realistic possibility a few years ago – the local marketplace hardly seemed big enough – is now a reality, as evidenced by the recent arrival of the joint-venture partnership chain Vets4Pets. This, according to Chris, is a real cause for concern and means that the local practice profession will need to be 'significantly more proactive' in their business dealings. Cromlyn recognizes that it has to both sustain its current client base and grow its business if it is to survive long term and 'ward off' local as well as corporate competition. Small-scale acquisition through the purchase of other small practices has been one of several business growth strategies explored by Cromlyn over the years; such practices could potentially act as 'feeders' to Cromlyn's Hillsborough base. Thus, by way of response to the corporate threat, toward the end of 2011 Cromlyn decided to open a branch practice in Lisburn (Hillsborough's nearest city). The new branch is located in an area of high visibility close to a roundabout and directly opposite the super-store Tesco. It is in a prime retail location, with its own customer parking. Opening the new branch made good business sense for Cromlyn who, while still considered a rural practice, have a growing Lisburn client base.

Meanwhile, back in Hillsborough, the Cromlyn team has finally been able to implement their long-standing plans to develop a specialist small-animal referral centre in an adjacent site. Having received the relevant planning permission, they have built two dedicated operating theatres. This is a significant business development for Cromlyn, with the new facility potentially being able to serve the entire NI small-animal sector and operate as a specialist, stand-alone business unit. Given the con-siderable resources required to develop such a spe-cialist service, and mindful of the fact that the NI market is relatively small, Cromlyn's new centre could well give the business a considerable compet-itive edge.

Another strategy adopted by Cromlyn to ward off corporate competition has been the introduc-tion of a pet health scheme. Their 'Pet Health Care Club' encourages clients to keep their pets' vaccinations up to date, allowing them to get dis-counts off other services. 'It's a sort of loyalty scheme, "locking in" clients' loyalty, with the ser-vice being offered when clients bring their pets in for their booster,' explains Chris. 'It's a way of offering a range of pet care services rather than a "one-off" consultation.'

Despite its relatively small size, the NI veterinary marketplace has recently become dynamic and highly competitive, and Chris will have to work hard to sus-tain his business of nearly 30 years. The arrival of Vets4Pets has essentially opened the door for further corporate expansion, promising big-brand presence secured in prime retail locations. Strategic small-scale acquisition or even green field site development to extend the Cromlyn brand are effective but highly expensive business strategies, and fully developing the new referral centre will take up most, if not all of Chris's time over the next 12 months.

As he prepares to see his first client of the day in the Hillsborough clinic, Chris starts to reflect on his *veterinary business journey* to date and thinks about the challenges ahead. He wonders how he can best secure Cromlyn's future and protect its position as an RCVS accredited hospital. Perhaps it is time to expand the partner team and get more support on the management side of the business? There may even be an opportunity to call on some of the younger team members for creative ideas – all interesting options for sure. Regardless of which strategy he chooses, Chris knows that Cromlyn needs to keep on moving forward, but where to now, exactly, he is not quite sure.

Acknowledgements

The author is extremely grateful to Chris Heffron, Managing Director of Cromlyn Vets, for his in-valuable input to the development of this case study.

References

Downes, M.J., Clegg, T.A., Collins, D.M., et al., 2011. The spatial distribution of pet dogs and pet cats on the island of Ireland. BMC Vet. Res 7, 28 (accessed 04.03.12). Available: http://www.ncbi.nlm.nih. gov/pmc/articles/PMC3141403/? tool=pubmed

Lantra, 2011. Veterinary activities factsheet, 2010–2011(accessed 03.03.12). Available: http://www. lantra.co.uk/Downloads/Research/ Skills-assessment/Veterinary-activities-v2-(2010–2011).aspx

PFMA, 2012. Pet Food Manufacturers' Association (accessed 19.10.12). Available: http://www.pfma.org.uk/ pet-population/

De'Ath, Slaughter, Davis & Jones, MsRCVS: time for a rebrand?

13

Lynne V. Hill

CASE OVERVIEW

This fictitious case study focuses on marketing and branding. It describes the various changes that have occurred to the caseload of an old, established rural veterinary practice, and discusses how the dynamics of the business have altered over the years. Based on feedback from the partners, staff, clients and referral practices, it is clear that several changes need to be made. The case explores whether a total rebranding is required and discusses the sorts of decisions that will need to be made in order for this to happen. The financial information provided in the case allows the reader to gain further insights into how the business has changed and determine the extent of the resources available to move forward.

LEARNING OUTCOMES

After reading this case study, students will be able to:
- Appreciate that the veterinary marketplace has changed and that client expectations need to be met.
- Understand the importance of getting practice feedback from both staff and clients.
- Draw on marketing and branding theories to make proposals that could help the old established rural veterinary practice depicted in this case study to deal with the changes to its caseload.

Introduction

It was a beautiful spring morning as John Davis, Senior Partner at De'Ath, Slaughter, Davis & Jones, walked his two Jack Russell terriers, Rinty and Jonty, across the Mendip Hills. This was John's favourite place to think, especially when he had tough decisions to make. During the 35 years he had spent in general practice in Somerset he had often drawn inspiration from the hills and beautiful views extending towards Glastonbury Tor and the Bristol Channel. He certainly had a problem now and needed to think about the way forward. The practice had reached a point where it needed to decide its future direction – to stay the same or to change? But not everyone was in agreement; John and Adam De'Ath wanted the practice to stick with its traditions and roots, while Mike Slaughter and Maggie Jones were pushing for a more modern marketing approach. The practice had recently invested in a new hospital on an out-of-town site and was about to move into its new premises, with the grand opening scheduled to take place in three months' time. However, a number of important issues still had to be resolved. For example, should the practice change its name? The consensus amongst the staff was that it should, and while a few suggestions for new names had been put forward, no firm favourite had yet emerged. How would the new hospital be advertised? While it was generally agreed to launch a marketing campaign, there was no marketing expertise in the practice. What about focus? Should the hospital stick to referral work or should it continue to include first-opinion services? It looked like this was going to be quite a long walk.

Practice history

The veterinary practice of De'Ath, Slaughter, Davis & Jones was first established in the city of Wells in the 1960s by John's grandfather, Charles; Charles

© 2014, Elsevier Ltd.

was later joined by John's father, James. Over the years, Charles and James built up a successful practice. They both retired, and three additional partners – Adam De'Ath, Mike Slaughter and Maggie Jones – joined the practice and, in 1985, they formed the current partnership of De'Ath, Slaughter, Davis & Jones.

The practice had initially developed to serve the farming community, located as it was in the heart of a strong dairy farming area. At the time, dairy farms were progressive, so it was important that the practice continued to serve them well during both the good and the leaner times. The practice became well established, developing a reputation for delivering prompt, effective service at a fair price.

By the late seventies, the practice had become a successful mixed practice, with the majority (around 80%) of the work being large animal. Small-animal work was carried out by all of the partners, but most of them preferred 'real' veterinary work with large animals.

Amongst the several changes witnessed by the veterinary profession in recent decades (see Box 13.1 for some additional background information), the gender shift is probably one of the most significant. The veterinary profession had traditionally been predominantly male dominated; however, by 1980, it started to undergo a rapid change through a significant increase in the number of women applying to vet schools. In 1975–76, 34% of graduates were female, but by 2005 this percentage had risen to 73%.

Box 13.1

Background information: some industry facts and figures

Current large-animal market

According to DEFRA (http://farmstats.defra.gov.uk), there has been a considerable decrease in the numbers of sheep, dairy and beef cattle over the last few years. Some of this has been as a result of disease outbreaks, such as foot and mouth in 2001. The number of farms continues to decrease, while herd sizes increase. Therefore, the need for the veterinary surgeon to supply a service for the single animal is generally in decline, and the new need is to provide a one-stop shop for the farmer through the larger framework of herd health planning.

Farm animal practice

There has been much consolidation in practices over the past few years as workloads have dropped, partners have retired and younger vets appear unwilling or unable to go into farm animal practice. Despite this, there are equally many examples of thriving farm practices in the southwest, e.g. Synergy Farm Health Ltd. and the Shepton Veterinary Group. However, it is no longer the case that farm animal clients will be satisfied with a 'fire brigade' service. It is essential to provide herd health planning, INTERHERD services and consultancy services in addition to the day-to-day care of animals registered with the practice.

Veterinary surgeon numbers

The number of veterinary surgeons in practice has risen from 8606 in 1996 to 10 399 in 2001, representing a 21% rise (RCVS/BVA/SPVS, Practice Survey 6, 2001). Total annual turnover of practices has risen from £1.07 billion to £1.45 billion over the same period – an increase of 35.5%. In 2011, 17 817 veterinary surgeons were registered on the 'practising register'.

Growth of referral practices

The number of referral practices in the UK has risen substantially in the past 5 years. Ten years ago most referral work was only provided by universities (six) and the Animal Health Trust (AHT). Interestingly, in the local area, the data suggest there is a consistency with the national trend. There are currently over 50 practices offering some type of specialized services within this case study practice's catchment area of 40 miles. In 2005, there were only 151 practices altogether in this area (RCVS Directory of Practices 2005). These figures demonstrate an expanding marketplace for veterinary services and an opportunity to increase market share for practices if the service offering is right.

One of the key factors in the recent expansion in the number of referral practices has been the growth in university-based qualifications. Universities have trained increasing numbers of postgraduate students, many of whom have taken up posts in private practices. The RCVS awards national certificates and diplomas, holders of which are eligible to become RCVS recognized specialists. In addition, there are specialist American and European colleges that award diplomas by examination. These also allow the holder to apply for specialist status.

The largest concentration of animals in the UK is found in the southeast, and the number of referral centres has been growing steadily in this area. This is now starting to have an impact on the southwest. Clients will travel long distances to ensure care at this level. Most competition in the southwest is from first-opinion veterinary practices with their own 'specialist' capabilities, often staff with certificate holders rather than diploma holders.

In 1983, Maggie Jones was the first female veterinary surgeon to join the practice. Despite the existing partners' and farmers' concerns about Maggie's ability to cope with large-animal work, she soon proved herself more than capable and quickly became a highly respected member of the team. John and Maggie got married in 1985 and had two children. Their daughter, Alison, also became a veterinary surgeon and was now working in one of the Australian universities, thus continuing the family tradition.

In 2000, the practice gained Veterinary Hospital status – the only one in the area at the time to achieve this, and currently one of a total of 165 in the UK (RCVS Facts 2011, https://www.rcvs.org.uk/publications/rcvs-facts-2011/). Although the partners were delighted, they did not think that they needed to change the way they did things, and the practice continued in much the same way as it had always done, without giving specific thought to its future identity or to the messages they were conveying to their clients or referring vets.

Following the foot and mouth disease outbreak in 2001, the practice lost a significant number of its farm clients. There was a subsequent decline in income from farm animal work, but income from small-animal work was starting to grow, as new housing estates were being built on the old farmland.

The present situation

The Hospital currently has a staff of ten vets (including the partners), fifteen nurses and five administrative staff. In addition to its first opinion work, it offers referral services to local practices. Referral work currently accounts for 25% of the practice's income. John had developed considerable expertise in cattle health and production, Maggie had a certificate in soft-tissue surgery and Mike Slaughter specialized in dermatology.

The practice has 150 active farm clients and around 10 000 small-animal clients. The majority caseload is small animal. Of the total £2.1 million revenue earned during the last financial year, just over £300 000 came from farm work, the majority of which was from drugs and medicines sales, as shown in the P & L account in Figure 13.1.

The steady growth that the practice has enjoyed over the past 30 years has slowed and is now less than 2%. The recession is starting to affect the Hospital's clients, with noticeably more people, particularly farm animal clients, experiencing difficulties paying their veterinary bills. According to one of the largest wholesalers in the veterinary industry, the veterinary market grew by less than 5% in 2010–11, and this growth is expected to fall further during the next 2 years. The Hospital's own data on active client numbers, average transaction values and income per vet reflect this continuing downward trend. In fact, revenues per vet, currently at £180 000 per annum, are at the lower end of the scale of average figures quoted in the SPVS surveys (Table 13.1).

Several new practices have recently set up in the area boasting new, modern premises and state-of-the-art equipment. One of these practices is now offering to provide out-of-hours services for other practices. As a Hospital, De'Ath, Slaughter, Davis & Jones are obliged to provide their own out-of-hours service, unless they can share with another hospital or a practice registered as an emergency clinic, as stipulated by the RCVS Practice Standards Scheme. In any case, John had always felt that the practice should do its own out-of-hours work, which is not always popular with the new recruits who do not wish to work at night for various reasons. John is beginning to wonder whether having Hospital status is actually an advantage, and does not really know how it is perceived by his clients.

The other partners have expressed concern about the increasing number of client complaints about costs, staff attitudes, opening times and the lack of adequate parking, although the parking situation will be greatly improved when the practice moves to its new premises.

The practice has also been losing staff, with two of the nurses leaving within the past 3 months, and another handing in her notice just a few days ago. It is not easy to find good nurses, and the costs of recruiting new staff are high. John wondered whether the practice was somehow 'putting off' applicants, either through its recruitment process, the level of remuneration offered or the overall impression the practice gives; jobs had been offered recently to two veterinary nurses, but both had turned them down.

The new young vets who had been appointed during the last 3 years appear to prefer small-animal work, even though they had claimed to enjoy large-animal work at interview. As a consequence, John carries out most of the farm work himself, with occasional assistance from the other vets, mainly at weekends, but is concerned that these vets are gaining little farm animal experience.

De'Ath, Slaughter, Davies and Jones

Trading and Profit and Loss Account for the Year Ending 30th April 2012

	2010		2011		2012	
Total revenue	1,881,601		2,060,040		2,100,820	
First Opinion	1,047,096		1,165,626		1,273,585	
Referral	435,377		502,314		525,205	
Farm	399,127		392,100		302,030	
Less Cost of Sales:						
Purchases (Drugs and consumables)	332,002	18%	362,600	18%	402,600	19%
Laboratory Fees	115,300	6%	121,520	6%	125,904	6%
Clinical Waste Disposal	10,500	1%	11,900	1%	12,600	1%
Casual workers/locums	14,500	1%	12,600	1%	15,800	1%
	472,302	1,409,298	508, 620	1,551,420	556,904	1,543,916
Gross Profit						
GP%	75%		76%		72%	
Less Administrative Expenses:						
TOTAL		1,093,827		1,150,831		1,260,048
Wages and salaries	993,567	53%	1,045,435	51%	1,152,000	55%
Rates and Water	9,540	1%	9,802	0%	10,200	0%
Light and Heat	11,980	1%	12,300	1%	12,500	1%
Insurances	10,500	1%	11,000	1%	12,000	1%
Property repairs	4,200	0%	6,000	0%	5,500	0%
Cleaning	6,500	0%	6,980	0%	7,500	0%
Telephone costs	5,410	0%	5,590	0%	5,609	0%
Postage and stationery	5,590	0%	5,912	0%	6,320	0%
Equipment hire	3,000	0%	3,000	0%	3,000	0%
Subscriptions	2,100	0%	2,250	0%	2,500	0%
Advertising	1,500	0%	1,500	0%	1,000	0%
Motor and travel costs	4,200	0%	4,500	0%	4,800	0%
Sundry expenses	4,530	0%	4,689	0%	4,598	0%
Accountancy Fees	5,500	0%	5,900	0%	6,200	0%
Bank and card charges	5,210	0%	5,223	0%	5,321	0%
Depreciation	20,500	1%	20,750	1%	21,000	1%
Net Profit (before interest and tax)		**315,471**		**400,589**		**283,868**
		17%		19%		14%

Figure 13.1 • Trading and profit and loss account

Table 13.1 De'Ath, Slaughter, Davis & Jones, MsRCVS: key performance indicators (KPI), April 2012

KPI	As at 30 April 2012
Active client numbers: small animals	10 000
Active client numbers: farm	150
Average transaction value (ATV)	£175[a]
Total number of transactions	12 000
Total revenue for year	£2 100 820
Income per vet (averaged)	£180 000

[a]Note that ATVs vary with different types of business, i.e. ATV farm = £270, ATV referral = £370, ATV first opinion = £39.

The partners' views

Maggie and John – Maggie and John had discussed these problems on a number of occasions, but had done little so far to address them. Maggie is in favour of a complete revision of the practice 'brand', but John is reluctant to let go of what he, his grandfather and father had built together, and is not convinced that a change would result in improved financial outcomes. Both agreed that they needed more information, and have decided to seek the views of both staff and clients through a series of one-to-one meetings with staff, and facilitated meetings with client groups.

Adam De'Ath – Adam is in favour of maintaining the status quo and cannot see why the practice needs to change. He is popular with the practice's small-animal clients and enjoys his work. Having reduced his hours to part-time last year, he is enjoying his hobby of sailing during his days off. Overall, Adam enjoys his life and is not inclined to support anything that might potentially disrupt this. In his opinion, the practice is simply not charging enough for its services. Seemingly, a speaker at a conference he recently attended in Florida, said: 'unless 10% of clients were complaining about the prices, the practice simply wasn't charging enough!' Adam had said as much to John, but John did not appear to be comfortable with the idea, so Adam did not pursue the issue.

Mike Slaughter – Mike is in agreement with Maggie. Most of his work at the practice is referral work, seeing dermatology cases, which he is good at and enjoys. But he also thinks that the practice could do much more and really should change with the times; it has been a 'traditional' practice for far too long. Secretly, Mike feels somewhat depressed about the lack of progress in his career since he joined as a relatively young partner in 1985, and unless things change he would seriously consider selling his share of the partnership and moving on.

John and Maggie asked the practice manager, Pat Hobbs, to organize a series of staff and client meetings, and these were held over the following month. John and Maggie urged the staff to be as truthful as they could when describing how they saw the practice and its future direction, and staff seemed to respond positively to being asked. The clients were delighted to be involved, as many of them had been clients of the practice for years and knew John and Maggie well. Pat Hobbs also made sure, however, that a number of new clients attended the meetings in order to obtain their opinions on why they had registered with the practice. Maggie also arranged to meet with referring vets to obtain their views.

The clients' views

Six weeks after the meetings with clients, Pat Hobbs and Maggie met to consider the feedback received. In general, the small-animal clients were satisfied with the quality of the veterinary care that was being provided, because most of their animals got better afterwards. However, apart from Maggie, Mike and John, the other vets were generally not very well liked. This appeared to be related to their poor communication skills, as well as their inability to explain things clearly, and the fact that they always seemed to be rushed and were unable to spare the time to talk things through properly. Clients also felt that the practice was badly in need of modernization. They were excited about the new premises and looking forward to bringing their animals there. The fact that some may have to travel a little further did not appear to be an issue, particularly since there would be ample parking.

The clients found the receptionists to be somewhat brisk, sometimes even rude, and did not show much empathy with them, but the nurses were perceived as hard working and very caring. There had been some problems with the computer system, as it was now quite old. It appeared to be very slow, and it often took too long to make an appointment, get an estimate or pay a bill. Clients felt that this, coupled with the long waiting times, needed to be improved.

The practice's farm clients were generally satisfied with the service provided, and John was a popular and respected vet. They were pleased to be able to see the same vet on every occasion, but felt that John was working much too hard and could not always manage on his own and needed help. They often had to wait a considerable time for him to arrive, which was both inconvenient and costly in terms of time wasted. They appreciated the reasonable prices that were charged, and John's expertise in herd health planning helped them to make considerable savings.

The referring vets' views

The words used by the referring vets to describe the practice were much more negative than expected. They said that the practice did not seem to care anymore, that it had become complacent and almost took it for granted that the work would come in. The receptionists provided a poor service, often failing to answer the phone or return their calls. The vets did not seem to have time to speak on the phone, or to give advice, and often failed to send their reports out in a timely manner. One referring practice said that on two occasions after an animal of a client had been put to sleep in the practice, they had not been informed and had to face the owners without this information, which was extremely embarrassing and unprofessional. As a result, this practice had decided not to send any more referrals to them. Similar messages were reported by several other referring practices.

The staff views

Pat Hobbs reported that staff morale was low. The vets felt they were working hard and delivering a good-quality service, but were being undervalued and had few opportunities for progression or to develop their skills and specific clinical interests. Most considered their jobs to be stepping-stones to other, better jobs in more progressive, modern practices elsewhere, and so were not as loyal to the practice as they could have been. The younger vets shied away from farm animal work, because John had little time to train them and, in any case, most farmers wanted John to attend because they knew him.

The nurses felt that they were also working very hard, but were not being fully appreciated or given the opportunity to develop their skills. They also felt that there was no point offering new ideas or suggestions for change, because the partners were too busy to listen and the other vets were always in a hurry and did not want to stay to talk about work after clinics were finished. The nurses felt that the practice should market itself more and pay more attention to clients' needs. They were keen to get involved in initiatives that would help strengthen the practice–client bond and improve team spirit within the practice. They also thought that the practice name was very cumbersome and old fashioned.

The receptionists complained of being overworked through having to serve both first-opinion clients and referring vets, whose needs were very different. They were unsure what the practice's priorities were because no one seemed to know. They often felt 'left out' of the information loop, and thought that appointing a head receptionist might help to address this.

The administrative staff were generally satisfied. They were all comfortable with their roles and could carry out their jobs with ease due to unchanged systems and procedures which, in their view, seemed to be working well. They also thought that from time to time the practice spent money unnecessarily and should look at making savings. However, they felt that the practice manager was easy to get on with, and was fair, kind and thoughtful.

The task ahead

Contemplating the feedback, John continued his walk across the fields and could just about spot Glastonbury Tor rising above the morning mist. The views of staff, clients and referring vets all made it clear that things had to change. It was time for a whole new identity – a new approach to doing business; big changes were needed. But John was starting to feel quite hopeful, because during his walk he decided that what the practice really needed was to hire a consultant – someone 'pretty clued up' on marketing and branding – to help the practice build a plan for the way forward. There were so many different directions the business could go, and working with the team to determine the most appropriate one for the practice would be the consultant's first priority. He called Rinty and Jonty to him and headed home.

Cascade Veterinary Practice: changing times

14

Adele Feakes   Diane Whatling

CHAPTER OVERVIEW

This case study explores the impact of poor management and changing demographics on Cascade Veterinary Practice, a mixed practice based in rural Australia. The veterinary partnership, owned by husband and wife team Tim and Mary Blake, is in serious difficulties as a result of their personal problems taking priority over the business, and there are no contingencies in place. The case shows how key performance indicators, as contained in the practice's extensive computer system, were ignored, and as a consequence the practice is in serious financial difficulty. The practice's issues are considered in light of both its internal and external operating environments. Although fictitious, this case scenario offers a valuable platform for identification and consideration of the opportunities for reinvigorating a floundering practice.

LEARNING OUTCOMES

After reading this case study, students will be able to:
- Understand the importance of monitoring key performance indicators in a veterinary practice.
- Appreciate the need to constantly monitor changes to the external environment.
- Apply business planning concepts to help offer potential solutions to salvage Cascade Veterinary Practice.

Introduction

Veterinarians Drs Tim and Mary Blake, husband and wife, own a rural veterinary practice in Cascade, rural Australia, and a small branch holding at Mandow, 25 km north. Both Tim and Mary are tiring of

veterinary practice and need a new lease of life, professionally and personally. Staff are concerned and at a loss as to what to do. Dr Dean Bletchley and Dr Tamara Savorio are veterinarians employed within the practice. Dean and Tamara have discussed the issue between themselves and have arranged to meet with the principal veterinarians to see if they can contribute to a solution. Tim and Mary have been great bosses for Dean and Tamara, and they really appreciate the support they have been given as new graduates. A preferred outcome would be that Tim and Mary would allow Dean and Tamara to get involved in the running of the practice and then they could take a well-earned break. Dean and Tamara feel up for the challenge; it could well open up opportunities for both of them, either by way of partnership or providing them with valuable experience for their own career paths.

Together, the four of them decided to meet on the Monday morning of the long weekend. Mary arranged with Kristy, a previous associate, to act as 'locum' that day so the full-time vets of the practice could get together. Kristy was fantastic like that, able to work from time to time as needed.

Background

Cascade Veterinary Practice is located in a rural area, although the town is undergoing urbanization. Small animal consultations are increasing and large animal call outs are decreasing. There are currently the two partner veterinarians (Drs Tim and Mary Blake), the two associate veterinarians (Drs Dean Bletchley and Tamara Savorio) and four nurses.

© 2014, Elsevier Ltd.

Seven years previously, the practice employed three veterinary associates and six nurses.

Tim and Mary met at veterinary school, married and graduated 25 years ago. After graduation, both Tim and Mary were keen to move chiefly into large-animal work but retain some small-animal work. They obtained their first veterinary positions in competing practices. After 3 years, they decided to purchase a large-animal practice of their own in a different area. The practice had been in existence for 24 years at the time Tim and Mary purchased it. It was a one-man practice and the veterinarian was looking forward to retirement. The practice, as a whole, was a 'good buy' back then, selling for $35 000 on 'goodwill' plus the Cascade building, which they purchased from the previous principal 6 months later. Tim and Mary struggled in the early days to make ends meet, with three young children and a sizeable loan with which they had financed the business and land purchase. Over the ensuing years, Tim and Mary made some improvements to the main clinic, which was originally a renovated bungalow. The changes were fairly minor, comprised of a new coat of paint, linoleum flooring, installation of office equipment and renewal of X-ray and anaesthetic machines.

To add to their main clinic in Cascade, Tim and Mary had purchased another building 15 years ago: a large shop (a former auction house) in the small town of Mandow, 25 km away. The practice only used rooms at the rear of the shop because the front parts of the building were tenanted. However, both tenants have recently vacated, leaving the main street frontage section empty.

Over the last 22 years, Tim and Mary grew the practice to five veterinarians (including themselves), four full-time nurses and two part-time nurses (all local people). However, now, the practice has just four full-time veterinarians: the partners and the two associate veterinarians, Dean and Tamara. These are supported by three full-time nurses and one part-time nurse. The full-time vets are each allocated a day a week to service the Mandow area, with Wednesdays covered according to booking demand. The Cascade clinic is open from 8.30 a.m. to 6 p.m. Mondays to Fridays, and from 9 a.m. to 12 noon on Saturday mornings. All the nurses work at Cascade. The Mandow premises are only open when the veterinarian is actually there, between calls or to take appointments; the Mandow clinic functions chiefly as a base for the veterinarian. Mandow, 25 km away, is serviced by a gently undulating, fairly straight and good bitumen road, such that the veterinarians can generally drive to Mandow in 25 minutes.

Dean, the older of the two full-time veterinary associates, has been in mixed practice for 4½ years and is quite 'comfortable' in his current work place. Dean spends his free time working in community groups and is planning to volunteer for a dog desexing programme overseas in the near future.

Tamara, who graduated 2 years ago, is developing into a very competent mixed-practice veterinarian, keeping herself busy studying for her membership of the Australian College of Veterinary Surgeons in Reproduction. She is very interested in reproduction in all common domestic species, and is particularly enjoying the work she is involved in with Tim, especially ultrasound pregnancy testing of horses, alpacas and goats.

The external environment

The profession

In the 1980s, Australian large-animal veterinary practices certainly 'rode on the back of the cow and the sheep', as did the Australian economy in general. With the Brucellosis and Tuberculosis Eradication Campaign (BTEC) and wool floor price schemes for the farmers around 1970–1990, cash flow was good for veterinary practices and wool producers, respectively. With the BTEC work, which was paid by the government, veterinarians regularly visited all cattle properties, so they knew their farm clients well. Cascade Veterinary Practice was a typical large-animal practice, which originated in the farming environment described above. Like many others, it had a generally casual approach to appointment scheduling, drug handling and providing free advice. Antibiotic resistance was virtually unheard of. Similarly, resistance to anthelmintic drenches was not yet recognized.

By the mid 1980s, brucellosis and tuberculosis were close to eradication in the more intensive livestock areas, so the need for private veterinarians to be harnessed into government paid work decreased. Then, around 1991, the wool 'floor price' was removed, and purchasing by the Australian Wool Corporation (AWC) for the stockpile was discontinued. This caused incomes to plummet for wool enterprises, the effects of which flowed on to businesses serving the farming community, including veterinarians.

Over the last decade or so, cattle and sheep prices have stayed relatively static, while costs of doing business have risen annually by at least the Consumer Price Index. Farming profits have narrowed, and farmers' core business now includes being 'land caretakers'. Farming enterprises are being sold to neighbours, so farming units are becoming much larger while still retaining the same level of management and labour units, thus becoming more efficient. In addition, for the last 2 years, eastern Australia has suffered several years of drought from a prolonged El Niño effect in the Pacific Ocean. As such, the local population of cattle and sheep has reduced to about 60% of previous levels. Now, in 2013, the Cascade and Mandow areas are entering a third year of drought.

The community

There are a number of other changes taking place within the Cascade and Mandow communities. Recently, a mining company – Eldanco – found valuable minerals in the surrounding area and has started to develop an infrastructure to support its business and worker population. Rural farming land and hobby farms around Cascade are now being purchased by Eldanco for exploration. Once a quiet rural area with a small village atmosphere, Cascade is quickly becoming a transport corridor for trucks. There is even talk of a rail system coming to town.

Currently, Cascade has a population of 26 000 residents, which is estimated to increase to 30 000 within 12 months, with a further 3000 inhabitants within 16 months. The population is a youthful one, with over half its residents aged between 18 and 44 years. There are insufficient rental properties and only enough schools to support the current population of children. Eldanco will have to fund much of the infrastructure to support employees and their families.

Cascade's unemployment rate is low, suggesting that outside labour will have to be brought into the town to fulfil Eldanco's workforce requirements. Many of the hobby farmers and rural holding farms are selling, as the prices offered for their properties are irresistible. Current prices for sheep and cattle are quite average, so with attractive offers on farm holdings these owners can see a way out of a plateauing industry. Some farmers wish to remain on the land and have purchased properties between 25 and 50 km north of Cascade, generally north of Mandow. These are the younger farmers who have a vision of cashing up and starting over with new herd

management techniques, new technologies and up-skilling in farm management. They can also see that the mining company will improve infrastructure such as shops and schools, and that this will be good for families even though they are 25 km or more away.

Mandow was, until recently, a sleepy little town with an ageing population of 730 people surrounded by large rural properties running sheep for wool and, more recently, alpacas. Many of the older Mandow farmers see the mining company as a blessing because they can sell their properties to Cascade farmers and retire. Twenty-five percent of current holdings are up for sale but are being rapidly sold for reasonably good prices. Change is coming for both towns, and this presents a real challenge for Tim and Mary in their approach to current rural veterinary practice.

Where did it all go wrong?

Nowadays, like many large-animal practices based in large country towns, Cascade is finding that small-animal consultations are increasing and large-animal call-outs are dropping. There are two other mixed veterinary practices within a 20 km radius south and east, both offering a reasonable service. Cascade's current combined client invoicing and patient history computer program allows analysis per species and client area. As such, the income from the clients of each branch and species group can be clearly seen in reports (Table 14.1, Figures 14.1 and 14.2). The mix of cases seen by the Cascade clinic compared to the Mandow branch has changed. At the time the computer program was installed, Cascade's income from large animals was similar to that from small animals. Initially, Tim and Mary were very keen to look at this sort of financial information, but over the last few years they have not been reviewing it in any great detail. Tim and Mary seem to be happy to just keep doing what they've always done.

Tim and Mary's business is in financial trouble, but it also has other problems in terms of leadership, operational controls, occupational and staff professionalism issues. The partners do not seem to be managing the business properly and currently Tim and Mary's personal problems seem to be taking priority over business issues. Strategic business planning based on actual facts and figures is badly needed, especially as the demographic and local economic environment is changing. Some sort of vision for the future is critical for both the Cascade and Mandow practices.

Table 14.1 Branch and species mix report

Period: 1/1/2012 to 31/12/2012	Large animals	Small animals	Total all species	%
Cascade	$93 758	$834 608	$928 366	67%
Mandow	$357 807	$95 286	$453 093	33%
Total practice gross income	$451 565	$929 894	$1 381 459	100%
%	33%	67%	100%	

This report shows the breakdown 'by income for each branch', 'by species mix for each branch' and also by species mix for the whole business. Note that the Mandow area brings in more than three times the large-animal work of the Cascade area.

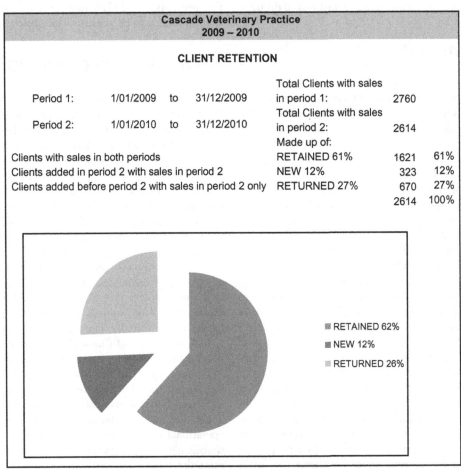

This table shows that client numbers were relatively static from 2009 to 2010, and that only 12% were new clients, 27% did not have any work done the year before but have returned, and 61% have had work done within this year and also in the year before (thus are "retained"). This analysis will differ depending on whether a practice is in a "growth" or a "plateau" phase. If the latter, then the practice would wish to see an increase in "retained" and a decrease in "returned" clients if customer service and marketing is working well.

Figure 14.1 • Client retention report

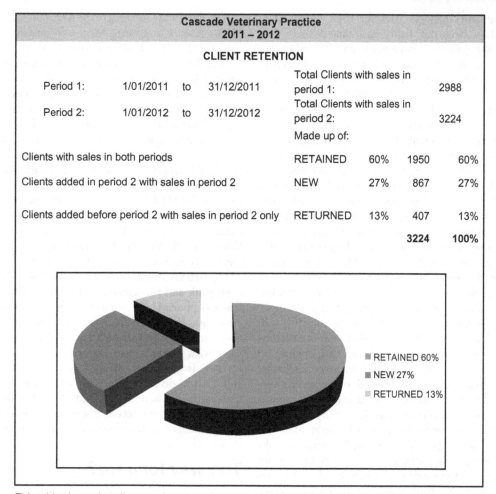

Cascade Veterinary Practice 2011 – 2012				
CLIENT RETENTION				
Period 1: 1/01/2011 to 31/12/2011	Total Clients with sales in period 1:			2988
Period 2: 1/01/2012 to 31/12/2012	Total Clients with sales in period 2:			3224
	Made up of:			
Clients with sales in both periods	RETAINED	60%	1950	60%
Clients added in period 2 with sales in period 2	NEW	27%	867	27%
Clients added before period 2 with sales in period 2 only	RETURNED	13%	407	13%
			3224	**100%**

■ RETAINED 60%
■ NEW 27%
■ RETURNED 13%

This table shows that client numbers have begun to grow from 2010 to 2012. Most importantly, the actual number of retained clients has increased from 2010.

Figure 14.2 • Client retention report

The physical state of both the Cascade and Mandow buildings is poor. Signage is particularly bad, and the overall image provided does not do justice to the high quality veterinary service that the practice actually provides for its clients. Equipment, however, is quite reasonable and has been maintained to a very good standard. Instrumentation, anaesthetic machines and monitoring equipment, radiology equipment, ECGs and ultrasound are all less than 5 years old.

Stock has slowly built up over the years in both the Mandow clinic and the mobile vehicles, and much of it is now expired. This was only discovered during an annual stock take in June. The Mandow premises are only staffed by the consulting veterinarian, with no nursing support, and often invoices are not paid before the client leaves.

Team morale is not particularly high, despite the practice having some dedicated long-term staff; two of the full-time nursing staff (Jane and Lyn) are eligible for long-service leave. The other full-time nurse (Lily) is pregnant. Tim and Mary wonder where they are going to get the money to pay the nurses when they take long-service leave, anticipating that this might happen sooner or later. Tim and Mary also worry about finding replacements for their experienced nurses. Current nursing staff have lower-level veterinary nursing certificates and have little ambition to develop their qualifications. Jane, one of the senior nurses, is on the verge of leaving because she cannot see any career development opportunities and is bored. Indeed, as well as failing to provide sufficient CPD (continuing professional development) opportunities for their nurses, Tim and Mary have not really maintained their own CPD, although they have made an effort this year as they need it for their registration. With regard to their other staff, Lyn, the second senior nurse, appears to be only there to collect a pay packet at the end of the week, and Lily is due to take maternity leave soon to have her first child. However, the part-time veterinary nurse, Susie, is enthusiastic, has excellent customer service skills and owns a successful part-time grooming facility run from home.

Cash flow is always tight, but especially this year, as many farmers have been paying their accounts as late as 6 months post invoicing. Farmers are having to pay enormous amounts for hay to be brought in due to the drought conditions, so are stretching out payments to their other creditors. Accounts and reminders are poorly managed in this practice. The appointment schedule has become patchy, especially after the last 2 years, which have been in drought. For example, on 2 days this week there have been only two call-outs to horses. All of this means that current cash flow is extremely poor and accounts are piling up (Table 14.3). Cascade's current veterinary wholesaler has cut credit, so they have moved to another one over the border. Mary has not taken a wage for 6 months (see Table 14.2), and this contributes to her stress as it undermines her feeling of worth. No matter how hard she works (see Table 14.5), it seems to make no difference; the profit and loss each month and for the last calendar year do not look too bad, but the overdraft just keeps getting bigger (see Tables 14.2–14.4).

Desperate measures

One night, at a real low, a very tired and run-down Mary looked at Tim and suggested that they actually consider closing the practice. It was obviously putting strain on their marriage and it had all become too much for her. Mary suggested she could not stand it any more and wanted to leave, not just the practice but Tim as well. Tim and Mary also talked about the impact of the mining company diminishing rural farms and their clients, concluding that all this would destroy them. Tired and depressed in the morning, Mary suggests she should leave Tim for a trial separation. The children are now 19, 20 and 22 years of age, and are all at university. The 22-year-old is in her last year of veterinary school, but is not sure what direction she would like to take with her veterinary career as yet.

Tim did not say anything to the rest of the staff about Mary's absence, suggesting Mary was going away to be with one of the children for a while. Three weeks went by and Tim became more and more depressed. He began drinking and refusing to take calls from clients. However, staff at Cascade Veterinary Practice eventually learned about Tim and Mary. Over the weeks Dean thought he had smelt alcohol on Tim's breath and observed some clumsy, inaccurate diagnosis and record keeping. Dean considered whether he should report Tim to the Veterinary Surgeons Board under the Medical Fitness to Practice provisions (Section 59 (1) (b)), but decided instead to talk to him about seeing his doctor and accessing the Australian Veterinary Association 24 hour Telephone Counselling Service maybe contacting the Australian Veterinary Association counselling service.

On two occasions during this period staff had not been paid, and this caused real friction. Tim's bank manager phoned him to make an appointment to discuss cash flow and the ever-increasing overdraft. Soon after, Mary returned from her 'supposed' break away with the kids, and she was clearly concerned for Tim. It was shortly after Mary's return that Dean and Tamara decided to ask for a meeting with the two partners where they could offer their support and indicate their interest in getting involved in the management of the business to help turn things around.

The way forward?

The discussion that ensued with Tim, Mary, Dean and Tamara on the Monday morning focused on identifying the main problems the practice was experiencing. Cash flow was high on the list, as were nurse staffing issues and the impact of the new mining company. Dean wanted to get Tamara more involved in the management of the practice; she was likeable, dependable, and a very competent and professional veterinarian. It would be difficult if Tamara decided to leave, as he would have to train another new graduate – not that he minded; it was just that Tamara was really 'firing up' as a veterinarian, and Dean enjoyed her professional input. Dean had no intention of leaving the practice as he was really enjoying the town and the community.

The four agreed that, as a starting point, they needed to gather all the facts and figures from the various reports available from the practice computer system, and take a hard look at the practice's performance before making any decisions (see all Tables 14.1–14.6).

Table 14.2 Income statement

Cascade Veterinary Practice – P & L Income Statement
Period: 1/1/2012 to 31/12/2012

GROSS INCOME (OPERATIONAL)

Total professional fees	$683 457	
Total drug and merchandise sales	$553 951	
Faecal egg counting in-house lab charge	$20 586	
Pathology – internal (15,544) and external (64,700) lab charge	$80 244	
Income – DETYA – trainee scheme	$5 500	
Travel total	$37 721	
Total income (or net sales) (or total operational revenues)		**$1 381 459**
Opening stock	$57 697	
Total purchases = medical ($221,156) + merchandise ($106,123)	$327 279	
Less closing stock	$74 755	
(Total) cost of goods sold (COGS)		**$310 220**
Total income – cost of goods sold = gross profit		**$1 071 239**

GENERAL EXPENSES (OPERATIONAL)

Pathology – internal ($10,556), external ($43,414) lab	$53 970
Imaging – radiology/ECG disposables, specialist referrals	$7 552
Experien X-ray processor lease	$3 376
Theatre – surgery costs – non-charged items	$15 700
Vet TB wage	$130 000
Vet MB wage	$70 000
Vet DB wages	$90 000
Vet TS wages	$77 500
Vet Superannuation guarantee @ 9% TB, MB, DB, TS	$33 075
Vet Sub-contract work – LOCUM (KS)	$11 922
Nurses – wages	$174 610
Nurses – superannuation @ 9%	$15 714

General employment expenses

Workers' compensation @ 1.75%	$6 745
Keyman Insurances DB	$1 236
Training, books, CE travel & accomm., AVA memb.	$16 388
Staff amenities, welfare, OHS, uniforms, prot. cloth	$10 011

Continued

Table 14.2 Income statement—cont'd

Promotional expenses	
Advertising and promotion (Yellow Pages)	$4 059
Printing, stationery and postage for advertising	$14 251

Facility and equipment expenses	
Rates	$8 607
Property repairs and maintenance	$17 022
Loose tool replacement and repairs to plant	$10 084
Computer software and maintenance	$5 221
Rubbish and body removal, cleaning and security expenses	$15 407
Electricity and gas	$11 807
Telephone, mobile, ADSL link, Internet	$11 425

Motor vehicle expenses	
Travel paid – veterinarians and nurses	$5 146
MV Holden utility lease Medfin	$8 904
MV Holden Utility fuel and oil, repairs and maint., reg., insurance	$8 945
MV Hilux SXR 786 interest*	$2 361
MV Hilux SXR 786 fuel and oil, repairs, reg., insurance	$5 234
MV Hilux SSR 786 depreciation	$6 026
MV Ford WNT 656 fuel and oil, repairs, reg., insurance	$2 730
MV Ford WNT 656 depreciation	$3 516
Hilux 2 SUV 007 lease Investec	$10 452
Hilux 2 SUV 007 fuel and oil, repairs, reg., insurance	$8 030
Animal transport interest*	$1 125
Animal transport repairs, maintenance, insurance	$1 666

Insurance expenses	
Insurance – land and buildings	$8 815
Prof. liability, public indemnity, S & A and business ins. TB MB	$12 099

Finance-related expenses	
Assets written off < $1 k	$2 648
Bad debts written off	$4 573
Bank charges and merchant fees	$8 283
Interest paid cheque account	$8 587
Interest paid credit Card	$2 841
Interest paid business loan	$8 601

Table 14.2 Income statement—cont'd

External consultants' expenses	
Accounting fees, legal and prof. fees	$16 234
Administration and miscellaneous fees	
Corporate registration	$3 960
Donations	$5 046
Freight and general postage	$4 053
Sundry expenses and petty cash	$1 822
Depreciation and amortization and depreciation low-value pool	$8 728
Bad debts expense and discounts allowed	$4 298
TOTAL GENERAL EXPENSES	**$980 405**
OPERATIONAL NET INCOME (OR LOSS)	**$90 834**
NON-OPERATIONAL INCOME AND EXPENSES	
Rent received	$6 761
NET INCOME (LOSS)	**$97 595**

This financial statement summarizes the income and expenses for a 'period of time'. This period of time is commonly either a calendar month (e.g. 1 May to 30 May), a 3-month period (e.g. a 'quarter', 1 January to 31 March, 1 April to 30 June, 1 July to 30 September, 1 October to 31 December), a calendar year (e.g. 1 January to 31 December) or a financial year (e.g. 1 July to 30 June [in Australia]). In Table 14.3, multiple equivalent terms have been used in places to familiarize readers with the various terms in use for the same thing. Similarly, abbreviations have been used, e.g. P & L stands for 'profit and loss'.

Table 14.3 Balance sheet

Cascade Veterinary Practice – balance sheet 31/12/2012	
ASSETS	
Cash	
Bank account	−57 591
Cash on hand, petty cash, change fund	723
Debtors	
Trade debtors/accounts receivable	**218 651**
Less: allowance for doubtful accounts	−9 556
Inventory	
Inventory merchandise stock and animal food	6 710
Drugs and medical supplies	64 050
Provision for slow/obsolete inventory	4 000
Prepayments and other assets prepayments	8 157

Continued

Table 14.3 Balance sheet—cont'd

Total current assets	**235 144**
Fixed (non-current) assets	
Land and building – Cascade	321 911
Land and building – Mandow	188 695
Furniture and fittings – Cascade	99 329
Accumulated depreciation – furniture and fittings	−37 800
Plant and equipment – high-value pool	90 175
Accumulated depreciation – high-value pool P&E	−60 852
Low-value pool	6 301
Accumulated depreciation – low-value pool	−5 290
Motor vehicles – Hilux SXR 786	54 813
Accumulated depreciation – MV Hilux SXR 786	−12 058
Motor vehicle Ford WNT 656	53 178
Accumulated depreciation MV Ford WNT 656	−46 146
Intangible assets goodwill	35 000
Total non-current assets	**687 256**
TOTAL ASSETS	**922 400**
LIABILITIES	
Accounts payable/trade creditors and accruals	
Accounts payable/trade creditors	91 058
Credit cards Diners and staff Mastercards	32 486
Current portion of long-term debt	3 600
GST – liabilities	
GST collected last quarter	55 000
GST to be paid for last quarter	−50 000
Payroll liabilities	
Annual leave provision	6 087
Provision for staff PAYG tax ($4087) and superannuation ($3003)	7 090
Total current liabilities	**145 321**
Business loan	94 929
Large-animal transport balance	12 778
Motor vehicle Hilux SXR 786 balance	51 097
Total long-term (non-current) liabilities	**158 804**

Table 14.3 Balance sheet—cont'd

TOTAL LIABILITIES	304 125
EQUITY	
Contributed equity partner TB & MB (50:50)	60 000
Drawings TB & MB	−670 000
Retained earnings	1 130 681
Current earnings	97 594
TOTAL OWNERS' EQUITY	618 275
TOTAL LIABILITIES AND OWNERS' EQUITY	922 400

This table shows the business's assets, liabilities and owners' 'equity' at a single point in time. Financial statements should be assembled relevant to a point in time, and the period preceding the point in time. This 'point in time' should ideally be at the end of a month, a 3- or a 12-month period.

Table 14.4 Transaction report

Cascade Veterinary Practice – transaction report
Period: 1/1/2012 to 31/12/2012

		Opening debtors' outstanding balance			$43,467.20
	Average $	No. of Invoices	Net $	Goods and services tax	Total $
NON-PATIENT INVOICES					
Settlement discount	−3.88	283	−99.17	−9.92	−109.09
Bad debt write-off	−505.62	13	−4573	−457.30	−5030.30
Adjusting journal	−4.96	18	−89.19	−8.92	−98.11
Voucher redemption	−57.51	4	−230.02	−23.00	−253.02
Rent*	813.33	12	6 761.00	676.10	7 437.10
Non-patient invoice totals	**$5.36**	**330**	**$1 769.62**	**$176.96**	**$1 946.58**
PATIENT INVOICES					
Consults – small animals	96.55	2 679	258 669.53	25 866.96	284 536.49
Prescriptions	96.35	3 092	297 898.76	29 789.88	327 688.65
Merchandise	36.86	2 183	80 474.20	8 047.42	88 521.62
Weight, nurse and NoChg	6.41	707	4 532.79	453.28	4 986.07
Vaccination	85.26	1 939	165 313.64	16 531.36	181 845.00
Farm visit	307.95	853	262 681.87	26 268.19	288 950.06
Euthanasia	49.70	153	7 603.99	760.40	8 364.39

Continued

Table 14.4 Transaction report—cont'd

Cascade Veterinary Practice – transaction report
Period: 1/1/2012 to 31/12/2012

	Average $	No. of Invoices	Net $	Goods and services tax	Total $
Surgery	294.37	252	74 181.76	7 418.18	81 599.94
Desexing	207.18	328	67 955.83	6 795.58	74 751.42
FEC including reports	60.32	309	18 639.78	1 863.98	20 503.76
Dentistry	251.18	57	14 317.52	1 431.75	15 749.27
Groom/clip	71.86	98	7 042.02	704.20	7 746.23
Hospitalization		459	43 841.99	4 384.20	48 226.19
Pathology	99.52	206	20 501.80	2 050.18	22 551.98
Work-up	157.90	366	57 794.08	5 779.31	63 572.36
Patient invoices totals	**$78.86**	**13 681**	**$1 381 449.56**	**$13 144.87**	**$1 519 593.43**
Patient + non-patient totals	**$72.93**	**14 011**	**$1 383 218.02**	**$138 321.80**	**$1 521 539.82**
			Sum (opening + invoiced)		**$1 565 007.02**
Payment – cash			$151 778.40		
Payment – cheque			$435 731.80		
Payment – Eftpos and credit card			$531 186.23		
Payment – direct debit			$227 659.90	**Total Receipted**	**$1 346 356.33**
			Closing balance of outstanding debtors		**$218 650.69**
			Change in unpaid balances		$175 182.39

This report is an example of a 'banking' report generated by a business's debtor program. The detail obtainable in such reports depends on the detail 'harvested' when creating invoices and receipts. This same report should be generated on a daily basis for daily cross-matching (or 'reconciliation') of the actual cash and electronic takings with the invoices and receipts ('debtors' program) for the day.

The practice's computer database certainly collected a significant amount of business and financial information, so perhaps it was high time they used it a bit more! All four agreed that the practice needed to work with the bank and their creditors, and focus on hauling in the debtors. Analysing the problems, identifying potential solutions and putting everything together in a strategic plan was going to be critical. The meeting drew to a close, with Dean and Tamara agreeing to meet again with Tim and Mary in a week's time to formally present their ideas. But this time the four would be joined by the bank manager. As Dean and Tamara left the meeting, they considered the incredible challenge ahead of them. How exactly were they going to turn things around?

Acknowledgements

This case study is fictitious. All persons, buildings, locations, and data used in this case study are not those of any real facility. RxWorks Veterinary Practice Management Software reports have inspired the layout of some of the tables.

Table 14.5 Product and service report

Cascade Veterinary Practice – product and services report – species: vet
Period: 1/1/2012 to 31/12/2012
(not including GST)

	Dr Tim Blake	Dr Mary Blake	Dr Dean Bletchley	Dr Tamara Savorio	Dr Kristy Sookie	Nurses – merchandise & FEC	Total $	Number of transactions	ATC
Alpaca	11 336	3 324	4 697	2 697	268	0	22 322	489	$45.65
Bird	303	403	503	133	93	623	2 058	87	$23.66
Cat	25 770	32 418	49 779	50 223	2 469	4 306	164 965	2 891	$57.06
Cattle	85 809	76 760	27 871	23 872	5 836	0	220 148	557	$395.24
Dog	158 093	166 397	216 389	183 675	8 090	18 540	751 184	7 915	$94.91
Donkey	1 066	1 266	2 156	1 956	0	0	6 444	60	$107.40
Ferret	88	0	389	89	470	101	1 137	23	$49.43
Goat	2 501	1 161	301	2 530	488	0	6 981	317	$22.02
Horse	20 068	19 664	20 068	27 201	10 073	3 413	100 487	557	$180.41
Sheep	30 052	40 686	13 952	11 952	1 752	6 789	105 183	689	$152.66
Wildlife	81	41	110	109	140	69	550	96	$5.73
TOTAL patient income	$336 167	$342 120	$336 215	$304 437	$29 679	$33 841	$1 381 459		
Transactions	2 486	2 750	3 233	2 063	250	2 899		13 681	
Average transaction charge (ATC)	$134.82	$124.41	$103.99	$147.57	$118.72	$11.67			$100.98

Table 14.6 Income group, medical and non-medical income report

Cascade Veterinary Practice – income group report

Period: 1/1/2012 to 31/12/2012

Dispensing fees	$30 615
Disposables	$1 586
Faecal egg counting	$20 586
Fleas and parasite	$78 090
Path/lab	$80 244
Prescription medicines	$381 408
Professional fees	$593 362
Travel	$37 721
Vaccinations	$44 701
Merchandise*	$100 604
Groom/clip*	$7 042
Department of Education and Youth Training Allowance	$5 500
Total OPERATIONAL INCOME	**$1 381 459**
Rent received	$6 761
Total all income	$1 388 219
MEDICAL × NON-MEDICAL INCOME REPORT	
1/1/2012 to 31/12/2012	
Total operational income	$1 381 459
Less non-medical Income*	−$113 146
Total medical income	$1 268 313

Items marked * contribute to non-medical income.

Northington Veterinary Clinic: a new lease of life?

15

Adele Feakes   Diane Whatling

CHAPTER OVERVIEW

This case study focuses on Northington Veterinary Clinic, a well-established and reputable small-animal practice based outside Adelaide, Australia. The practice premises have not been maintained or upgraded over the years. The principal veterinarian, Peter, is considering retirement. The business needs a new lease of life, so both a renovation and succession plan are urgently required. This fictitious case study provides students with valuable insights into veterinary practice management, highlighting potential problems that can arise when a practice fails to keep up to date with equipment, financial management and premises, or simply does not avail itself of potential development opportunities.

LEARNING OUTCOMES

After reading this case study, students will be able to:
- Appreciate the importance of updating practice premises and keeping up to date with changes in the external environment.
- Understand the need to manage and act on critical practice performance information.
- Apply business concepts to develop a strategy outlining the way forward for Northington.

Introduction

Northington Veterinary Clinic (NVC) is situated on the edge of the city business district of Adelaide, South Australia. Dr Peter O'Connor, the principal and owner, has reached 50 years of age; he is somewhat tired of working full-time and is contemplating retirement. Dr Jim Chew, his associate, on the other hand, is only 30 years of age and needs to work on developing both his career and his assets. Jim is really keen to develop the practice and sees lots of exciting opportunities that can be pursued, but is mindful that the practice has become run down over the years, and that this needs to be addressed before the business can move forward.

Peter and Jim have both returned from their respective holidays eager to look towards the future. Although from two different generations, they are good friends and colleagues and both want the best for the practice (and themselves). They agree that they should sit down together to decide on the best course of action to provide NVC with a 'new lease of life'.

Background

NVC is housed in an old-style building on a busy road with adequate parking. It has been a veterinary icon in the area for 24 years, with its distinct traditional blue vet sign taking up much of the street frontage aligned with the footpath. In its early days, NVC was recognized as one of the better veterinary practices in the area, with separate operating rooms and expansive cage areas. The waiting room, though small, was bright and well kept. Signage was innovative for the time. However, now the building is looking tired and the signage is old; there is graffiti on the side of the building, giving it an unkempt appearance. There are no windows to the front, just a brick wall with ivy overgrowing the signage, and a standard wooden door for the main entrance.

© 2014, Elsevier Ltd.

The small waiting room has four wooden benches attached to the wall. It has been 10 years since the walls were painted. There is a stand with a few shampoos and brushes, none of which are priced, and there is no product information available to clients, bar a few pamphlets on vaccinations. Practice business cards or additional information are rarely provided to clients.

The consulting room walls are painted a traditional white, and there is a stark stainless steel table with painted legs centrally located, and a bench against the wall with a few instruments. All medications are dispensed from the consulting room, including dangerous drugs that are kept in cupboards with doors in need of repair. There is a second consulting room, but this is currently used as a storage area. The preparation area for surgery is small, but the hospital area for holding pets is huge. There is also a surgical theatre that is well lit but is in need of refitting. Unfortunately, the operating theatre has a two-way entry system, causing issues with sterility and airflow. Disappointingly, the theatre has not been upgraded with new technologies; for example, there is no anaesthetic monitoring equipment in place.

External environment

The profession

The ever-increasing use of technology has certainly impacted on the veterinary profession. Veterinarians have to keep up with medical advancement, new drugs, equipment and techniques. Purpose-designed, built and furnished practices are starting to appear along with a new generation of vets. Some parts of the profession realize that a veterinary business is actually like other any business – one that requires management, monitoring, care, financial accountability, marketing and an entrepreneurial approach. Practice managers, until very recently, were brought across and adapted from other professions and businesses, and generally came from a financial management or human resources role. Veterinary practice management courses are now available, and groups within the profession have begun benchmarking against each other.

In the 1970s, legislation for professional advertising changed to allow professionals such as veterinarians, dentists, doctors and lawyers to advertise

their business. At first, these professionals were guarded about advertising, essentially due to having no training in marketing. Some veterinarians identified opportunities to develop a competitive edge and entice clientele to their practices. Initially, poor marketing ideas were used. For example, Yellow Pages advertising in the telephone book used to be seen as the ultimate marketing tool. The use of external signage and visual identity was also new to the profession. Murals, neon signs and large print appeared on buildings; some were quite effective, but others were inappropriate or difficult to read. More recently, internet and social media have also become important for brand awareness and advertising, but there is still a wide range of variation in the profession in achieving effective social media presence.

The community

NVC is located in a leafy green suburb 5 km from Adelaide's' central business district (CBD). Northington itself has a population of 36 000 people in 15 000 households, and the population is increasing at 5% per annum. Community land use is predominantly residential, with some commercial areas. The suburb is undergoing a cyclic demographic change. The population was, until recently, predominantly aged, but now 42% of the population is between 35 and 49 years.

Professionals and managers are over-represented in the local area, being 36% and 15.6% of the population, respectively, as compared to 20.5% and 11.4%, respectively, for Adelaide overall. Therefore, disposable income is likely to be above average. The younger people moving into the Northington area are renovating and refurbishing older houses. Although Northington's population is increasing, the local council is keen to maintain its village and heritage image.

Dog and cat ownership levels are difficult to determine, as dog registration is the only statistic recorded by the council. Estimated figures suggest that only 63% of dogs are registered. The council finds it difficult to administer dog registrations, and the cat population is unknown. There are dog parks, and generally the council receives few complaints regarding barking dogs and dogs wandering at large. The town of Northington has a well-designed Animal Management Plan in place for the next 5 years, which permits a maximum of two dogs per household. Micro-chipping will soon become mandatory for dogs and possibly cats, along with cat registration. Northington Council, in conjunction with a neighbouring vet practice, provides education programmes to the public about responsible pet ownership.

The problem

NVC is in serious need of renovation. When Peter's parents supported its inception in 1988, the practice was innovative and state of the art. Peter, the practice principal, was enthusiastic and wanted to practise excellent veterinary medicine. He started the practice with just himself and two untrained part-time veterinary nurses. Two years later, he employed Marge, the practice manager.

Peter enjoyed going to conferences to keep up to date with new clinical developments and catch up with colleagues from his university days. When Peter was away, Marge, along with the two nurses and locums, ran the business. However, Peter noticed that while he was away the practice income reduced by half. This prompted Peter to employ his first associate back in 1993.

Dr Jim Chew was employed as a new graduate in 2007. Jim is a progressive, visionary veterinarian with a special interest in orthopaedics and general surgery. Dr Sue Smith subsequently joined the practice in 2010 as an associate, working part time as she has two young children. Sue is a very competent veterinarian, with 8 years' experience, and has a special interest in feline medicine and pocket pets. Peter, the owner, while an average all-round clinician, has run the practice over the years with 'peaks' and 'troughs' of energy. However, over time, the 'peaks' have become smaller and the 'troughs' have become bigger.

Marge, the practice manager, has always been very keen on her role but it was clear from the very start that she lacked skills. For example, she is strong in financial reporting and administration, but somewhat deficient in human resource management. Marge believes continuing education is a waste of time for nurses and that the only skill a nurse should have is a good holding technique so that the vet does not get bitten!

Hayley and Fiona are full-time veterinary nurses in their mid-twenties, each only at the level of the first Certificate of Veterinary Nursing. Fiona is the newer of the veterinary nurses, having been with the practice for 12 months. There has been little encouragement to undertake further training in veterinary nursing, and the nurses have limited personal motivation to do so. Their main job description is to answer the telephone and to clean. This frustrates the two younger vets, who try to encourage an ethos of good practice protocols.

A taxing time

Late in 2012, Peter was audited by the taxation department for not paying Goods and Services Tax (GST), but in fact it was Marge who had not done so. Peter received a $12 000 fine and now has to pay back payments of $53 000 to the taxation department. Small amounts of money have also gone missing. A daily reconciliation of transactions is kept but it rarely balances. Different clients come in each month, as they have been getting accounts in the mail, but claim that they have already paid (see Tables 15.2 and 15.3).

Although he is the practice owner, Peter does not consider details such as the income statement, fee schedules, staffing budgets and service reports as important. As long as there is a small amount of money in the bank to support his annual holiday and conference then he is satisfied. However, the clinic's income has plateaued over the last 18 months, and since the taxation debacle cash flow has been especially poor. Fortunately, Marge maintains the debtors, creditors and general ledger systems adequately for extraction of information to go to both the accountant and, on occasion, into a practice benchmarking service. This practice benchmarking service enables a practice to compare its key financial performance indicators to other similar Australian veterinary practices. NVC's software program also allows further custom reports that include further species and transaction analysis (see Tables 15.1–15.8 and Figure 15.1).

Managing clients

Over the years clients have remained loyal to Northington, despite the practice being inconsistent in providing vaccination, check-up or follow-up reminders. During the last decade, two major competitors have established modern progressive veterinary clinics within a 5 km radius but this does not seem to worry Peter, as he believes his bedside manner and cheaper prices will maintain his client base.

Peter has actually increased fees for the past 2 years, but he himself continues to charge what he thinks is appropriate for some clients (see Table 15.1).

Table 15.1 Products and services report by species by vet or staff member

Northington Veterinary Clinic

Products and services – species: vet or staff

Period: from 1/1/2012 to 31/12/2012

	Dr Peter O'Connor			Dr Jim Chew			Dr Sue Smith			Staff sales			Total
	Charged	No.	Avg.	Charged	No.	Avg.	Charged	No.	Avg.	Charged	No.	Avg.	Total $
Bird	$220.64	399	$0.55	$2 045	47	$43.51	$957.53	32	$29.92	$418.00	150	$2.79	$3 641.17
Cat	$55 537.90	1190	$46.67	$127 332	1290	$98.71	$41 617.03	420	$99.09	$1 492.70	303	$4.93	$225 979.63
Dog	$321 841.60	3500	$91.95	$337 228	2011	$167.69	$48 474.68	504	$96.18	$2 627.90	402	$6.54	$710 172.18
Small pets	$5 812.30	160	$36.33	$5 070	508	$9.98	$5 367.89	80	$67.10	$575.30	206	$2.79	$16 825.49
Wildlife	$66.72	46	$1.45	$64	61	$1.05	$0.00	51	$–	$ 286.00	104	$2.75	$416.72
	$383 479	5295	$72.42	$471 738	3917	$120.43	$96 417	1087	$88.70	$5 400	1165	$4.64	$957 035.19

Table 15.2 Invoices, balances and banking transaction summary report

Northington Veterinary Clinic

Financial report – by type of transaction

Period: from 1/1/2012 to 31/12/2012				Opening balance: debtors at 1/1/2012		$12 797.15
Non-patient invoices	**Average amount**	**No. trans.**	**Net**	**Tax**	**Total**	
Settlement discount	−34.10	1	−34.10		−37.51	
Bad debt write-off	−291.54	7	−1,855.27	−185.53	−2 040.80	
Adjusting journal	−27.25	282	−6 985.97	−698.60	−7 684.57	
Account fee	2.52	372	853.50	85.35	938.85	
Total non-patient invoices	*−$13.33*	*662*	*−$8 021.84*	*−802.18*	*−$8 824.02*	
Patient invoices						
Professional fees	103.70	5 857	552 163.08	55 216.31	607 379.39	
Drugs and prescription food dispensed	102.16	4 060	377 071.75	37 707.18	414 778.93	
Accessories and non-prescription food	8.36	264	2 007.50	200.75	2 208.25	
Weight check	2.94	102	272.35	27.23	299.58	
No charge	0.00	878	–	0.00	0.00	
House visit	47.42	8	344.89	34.49	379.38	
Pathology	93.87	295	25 174.88	2 517.49	27 692.36	
Total patient invoices	*$91.83*	*11 464*	*$957 034.45*	*$95 703.45*	*$1 052 737.90*	
Total patient and non-patient invoices		*12 126*	*$949 012.61*	*$94 901.26*	*$1 043 913.88*	*$1 043 913.88*
			Sum opening balance + invoiced in period =			$1 056 711.03
Payment – cash		205 427.20				
Payment – cheque		38 933.52				
Payment – EFTPOS		248 886.20				
Payment – credit card		472 780.60				
			Total receipted in period			$966 027.52
			Closing balance debtors at 31/12/2012			$90 683.51
			Change in unpaid balances over the period			$77 886.36

Table 15.3 Invoices, balances and transactions: type of client

Northington Veterinary Clinic

Balance and transactions – by type of client
Period: from 1/1/2012 to 31/12/2012

Account type	Total clients	Active clients	No. of invoices	Opening balance	Invoiced	Payments	Closing balance
Bad debt	171	41	185	10 225.25	9 629.09	7 670.55	12 183.79
Cash only	307	207	957	1 116.34	72 486.32	65 642.00	7 960.66
Normal	17 909	2959	12 594	785.46	867 096.76	808 214.18	59 668.04
Public trustee	3	1	26	−182.1	1 554.14	981.19	390.85
Staff	25	13	349	295.8	7 187.41	6 511.45	971.76
Valued	43	23	733	556.4	85 960.15	77 008.15	9 508.40
	18 458	3244	14 844	$12 797.15	$1 043 913.86	$966 027.52	**$90 683.50**

Northington Veterinary Clinic **Client Retention Report**

Period 1:	1/01/2011	to	31/12/2011	Total Clients with sales in period 1:		2988	
Period 2:	1/01/2012	to	31/12/2012	Total Clients with sales in period 2:		**3224**	

Clients with sales in both periods	RETAINED	60%	1950	60%
Clients added in period 2 with sales in period 2	NEW	27%	867	27%
Clients added before period 2 with sales in period 2 only (and not in period 1)	RETURNED	13%	407	13%
			3224	**100%**

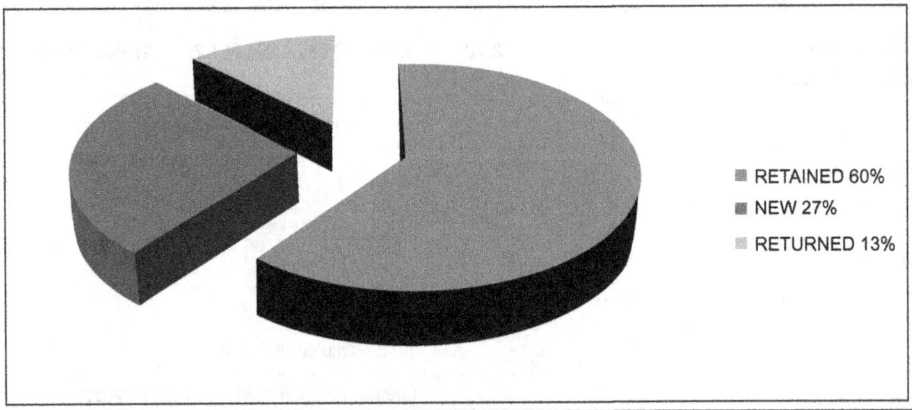

This figure shows the client numbers for the two whole year periods for 2011 and 2012. 60% have had work done in both years (thus are "retained"), 27% were new clients, and 13% did not have any work done in 2011 but have returned. This analysis will differ depending on whether a practice is in a "growth" or a "plateau" phase. If the latter, the new clients would be stable from year to year around a lowish figure, while the practice would wish to see a high percentage in "retained" and a decrease in "returned" clients if customer service, marketing and wellness programs are working well.

Figure 15.1 • Client retention report

Table 15.4 Income–expenses statement (profit and loss)

Northington Veterinary Clinic	
Income–expenses statement 1/1/2012 to 31/12/2012	
INCOME (FROM SALES) ALSO KNOWN AS 'REVENUE'	
Total professional fees	$544 758
Drug sales	$377 072
Pathology – companion animal	$25 175
Accessories, dog food and non-medical sales	$2 008
TOTAL (NET) SALES ALSO KNOWN AS TOTAL PRACTICE REVENUE (TPR)	**$949 013**
Opening stock	$37 657
Purchases – drugs and medical supplies	$303 478
Purchases – accessories, dog food and non-medical	$1 453
Less closing stock	$48 354
COST OF GOODS SOLD	**$294 234**
(= opening stock + purchases – closing stock)	
GROSS PROFIT	**$654 779**
(= total sales – cost of goods sold)	
GENERAL EXPENSES (INCURRED TO ACHIEVE SALES)	
Pathology	
External laboratory	$18 309
Imaging	
Radiology, monitoring and imaging disposables	$1 741
Ultrasound – visiting ultrasonographer, referral fees	$400
Wages and salaries expenses	
VETERINARIANS	
Wages – JC	$95 000
Wages – SS	$38 000
Superannuation guarantee salaried vets @ 9%	$11 970
Owner's 'salary' (note, in this case is taken as a drawing so not shown in income/expenses statement)	$0
NON-VETERINARIAN: MANAGEMENT AND ADMINISTRATION	
Wages	$44 249
Superannuation guarantee @ 9%	$3 982
NON-VETERINARIAN EMPLOYEES (NURSES)	
Wages	$58 716

Continued

Table 15.4 Income–expenses statement (profit and loss)—cont'd

Northington Veterinary Clinic

Income–expenses statement 1/1/2012 to 31/12/2012

GENERAL EXPENSES (cont.)

Superannuation guarantee @ 9%	$5 284
NON-VETERINARIAN EMPLOYEES (OTHER THAN NURSES)	
Wages – casual	$1 744
Superannuation guarantee @ 9%	$0
General employment expenses – all staff	
Workers compensation @ 1.75%	$4 532
PO'C sickness and accident insurance	$3 612
Books and journals, staff/vet CE, prof. memberships	$7 972
Staff amenities and welfare and OHS	$3 510
Staff uniforms/laundry	$1 569
Groomers' commissions	$1 929
Promotional expenses	
Advertising and promotion	$175
Yellow Pages	$4 606
Printing and stationery	$3 900
Facility and equipment expenses	
Land rates and water rates	$10 280
Building Lease O'Connor Trust	$52 383
Repairs and maintenance – building	$2 830
Repairs and maintenance equipment	$4 453
Rubbish removal and body disposal	$11 510
Cleaning expenses	$3 343
Electricity and gas	$6 929
Telephone, Internet access, alarm	$9 680
Other IT and veterinary software maintenance	$3 496
Motor vehicle repairs and maintenance, fuel and oil	$1 182
Travel	$685
Insurance expenses	
Insurance – land and buildings	$4 261
Insurance – motor vehicles	$859
Professional liability insurance	$5 651

Table 15.4 Income–expenses statement (profit and loss)—cont'd

Northington Veterinary Clinic

Income–expenses statement 1/1/2012 to 31/12/2012

GENERAL EXPENSES (cont.)		
Finance-related expenses		
Debt collection	$2 451	
Bank charges and fees	$8 634	
Interest paid to bank – overdraft	$786	
Interest paid to bank – variable loan	$6 883	
Interest HA & IS O'Connor Loan	$850	
External consultant expenses		
Accounting fees	$5 643	
Legal and professional fees	$14 307	
Administration and miscellaneous expenses		
Donations	$3 216	
Freight and postage	$5 741	
Depreciation and amortization	$12 725	
Petty cash expenditure	$1 265	
TOTAL GENERAL EXPENSES		**$491 243**
NET OPERATING INCOME (LOSS) (= gross profit less total general expenses)		**$163 536**
OTHER INCOME/LOSSES		
Interest income	$0	
Other Income, e.g. gain on sale of investment	$0	
Other expenses and losses	$0	
Loss on sale of equipment	$0	
NET INCOME (LOSS) BEFORE INCOME TAXES		**$163 536**

This financial statement summarizes the income and expenses for a 'period of time', which may be for example a calendar month, a 3-month period (e.g. a 'quarter', 1 January to 31 March), a calendar year (e.g. 1 January to 31 December) or a financial year (e.g. 1 July to 30 June in Australia). In the above, multiple equivalent terms have been used to show the various terms and abbreviations in use for the same thing.

This causes issues with other staff, especially Jim. Dispensing fees and injection fees are low or non-existent and, overall, the average drug mark-up achieved is only 28% (use Table 15.4 to calculate this). Drugs are dispensed in envelopes with hand-written labels that are barely legible. The drug store contains expired drugs, especially injectables, some of which are out of date by 2 years or more. Many medications, including shampoos, are bottled in refillable clear plastic bottles, with simple labelling and directions.

Table 15.5 Fee schedule

Northington Veterinary Clinic

Schedule of fees @ 1/7/2012

Consultation normal		$53.50
Consultation revisit or 2nd animal		$42.50
Prescription fee		$6.00
Injection fee (per injection)		$5.50
Dog annual health check and vacc.		$83.95
Cat annual health check and vacc.		$73.95
Cat spey (add 25% for advanced pregnancy)		$169.50
Cat castration		$104.00
Dog spey < 10 kg (add 25% for advanced pregnancy)		$247.00
10–25 kg (add 25% for advanced pregnancy)		$307.00
25–45 kg (add 25% for advanced pregnancy)		$407.00
Dog castration < 10 kg		$187.50
> 10 kg		$227.50
Radiographs first plate		$102.50
Second and further plates		$55.40
Anaesthetic, local or light sedation		$27.00
Heavy sedation – cat or dog		$87.00
General < 30 min		$118.00
Per hour		$151.00
Surgery hourly rate		$302.00
Theatre fee		$40.00
Hospitalization	24 hours (standard care)	$30.50
	Per 24 hours (on IV fluids)	$107.00
Fluid therapy	IV set-up and first litre with infusion pump	$107.00
	Subsequent litres	$20.50
Dentistry	20 min scale and polish only (add GA and meds)	$149.40
	60 min procedure incl. extractions (add GA and meds)	$400.00
Lab in-house	Urinalysis, S.G. and dipstick	$16.50
	Sediment examination, cytology, skin scraping, FNA or impression smear	$30.75
	PCV/total protein or single in-house biochem. (e.g. urea)	$20.00

Table 15.5 Fee schedule—cont'd

Northington Veterinary Clinic

Schedule of fees @ 1/7/2012

Pre-anaesthetic biochemistry profile (e.g. in-house)	$63.60
Haematology (e.g. in-house)	$23.00
Full biochem. profile (e.g. in-house)	$98.20
External lab fees mark-up %	20.00%

Table 15.6 Neighbouring clinics' fees (per phone calls made)

	North Road Clinic	Tail Wagger Clinic
Consultation normal	$57.50	$60
Dog annual health check and vacc. (C5)	$85	$87.50
Cat annual health check and vacc.	$75	$77.50
Cat spey	$190	$220
Cat castration	$100	$140
Dog spey 7 kg	$275	$350
16 kg	$350	$400
28 kg	$450	$450
Dog castration <7 kg	$225	$247.50
> 25 kg	$290	$300

Table 15.7 Balance sheet

Northington Veterinary Clinic Balance sheet – 31/12/2012

Current Assets

Working bank account	$1 632	
Cash on hand, undeposited funds, petty cash, payroll ACC	$15 967	
Debtors/accounts receivable	$90 684	
Less: allowance for doubtful accounts	−$18 657	
Pre-payments and other assets	$6 473	
Total cash and receivables		$96,099
Inventory drugs and medical supplies	$45 133	

Continued

Table 15.7 Balance sheet—cont'd

Northington Veterinary Clinic Balance sheet – 31/12/2012

Inventory animal food	$3 221	
Total inventory		*$48,354*
Total current assets		**$144 453**
Fixed (non-current) assets		
High-value pool plant and equipment (P&E)	$115 633	
Accumulated depreciation – high-value pool P&E	−$76 162	
Furniture and fittings (F&F), computer hardware	$25 000	
Accumulated depreciation – F&F, computer hardware	−$23 333	
Land and buildings (at original cost)	$143 454	
Building development 1996	$178 457	
Motor vehicles – Hyundai	$53 178	
Accumulated depreciation – MV	−$2 511	
Low value pool	$2 925	
Intangible assets – goodwill, trademark/registered logo	$0	
Total fixed assets		**$416 641**
TOTAL ASSETS (CURRENT AND FIXED)		**$561 093**
Current liabilities		
Accounts payable/trade creditors	$31 057	
Diners Club & Business Mastercard PO'C	$32 302	
Current portion of long-term debt	$2 050	
Net GST (collected − paid) previous quarter, owed to tax office	$11 174	
Provision for annual leave and long-service leave	$5 282	
Other liabilities		
Outstanding taxation (PO'C) and fines (PO'C)	$65 000*	
Total current liabilities		**$146 865**
Non-current (long term) liabilities		
Variable-choice loan conversion	$10 430	
HA & IS O'Connor loan – interest only	$10 000	
Hyundai chattel mortgage balance	$49 178	
Hyundai unexpired interest	−$1 547	
Total non-current liabilities		**$68 061**
TOTAL LIABILITIES (CURRENT AND NON-CURRENT)		**$214 926**

Table 15.7 Balance sheet—cont'd

Northington Veterinary Clinic Balance sheet – 31/12/2012

Owners' equity (net assets)

Contributed capital owner	$300 000
Net income	**$163 536**
Drawings	-$513 420
Retained earnings	$396 051
	$346 167
TOTAL LIABILITIES AND STOCKHOLDERS' EQUITY	**$561 093**

This table shows the business's assets, liabilities and the owners' 'equity' at a single point in time, ideally at the end of a month, a 3- or a 12-month period.

Table 15.8 Benchmarking reports – key performance indicators

Profitability and activity ratios

Measure	Equation
Return on sales	Net income/revenue from sales i.e. Total Practice Revenue (TPR)
Inventory turnover (IT)	Cost of goods sold/average inventory
Inventory days in stock	365/IT

Productivity ratios

FTEs of veterinarians	Total hours worked all vets/38
Average revenue per vet	Total practice revenue 'TPR'/FTE vets
Medical revenue per vet	Total non-medical revenue/FTE vets
Average transaction charge (ATC)	TPR/total no. of transactions
Medical average transaction charge	Total non-medical revenue/total no. of transactions
Annual no. of transactions (invoices) per vet	Total no. of transactions per year/FTE vets
Active clients per vet	No. of owners visiting in last 12 months/FTE vets
New clients per year per vet	No. of new clients in year/FTE vets
Annual transactions per client	Total no. of transactions in year/no. of active clients
Average annual revenue per client	TPR/no. of active clients that year

Cost control KPIs

Drugs/medical supplies as % of revenue	Total cost of drugs and medical supplies/TPR
Laboratory costs as % of revenue	Total lab costs/TPR
Retail product expense as % of revenue	Total OTC costs/TPR
Non-vet wages and benefits as % of revenue	Total support staff costs (plus on-costs)/TPR
Rent as % of revenue (maybe notional)	Total rent/TPR
Total costs as % of revenue	Total costs/TPR

An unfortunate event

Treatment plans are changed on a regular basis by Peter when he picks up another veterinarian's case. This causes friction, and in one case led to an investigation by the Veterinary Surgeons Board. This particular case involved a 1-year-old, female Border Collie called Jess. Jess had been seen by Jim initially on a Friday night. The dog presented with lethargy, inappetance, fever and some minor abdominal pain in her caudal abdomen. He was suspicious that Jess had an infected uterus, although no vaginal discharge was present. The X-ray machine was not working; Marge had promised to phone a technician several days ago but had not done so. Jim administered injectable antibiotics and strongly requested the owner to return with Jess the next morning for a revisit consultation. Jim left detailed notes outlining Jess's problem list, possible diagnoses and treatment plan. He had calculated dose rates of antibiotics, noting in large print that Jess had a temperature of 40.0° C.

Peter was consulting on Saturday morning. The last patient of the morning was Jess. The owner reported that there was no improvement in Jess's condition; in fact, Jess appeared worse. Peter asked the owner if she had eaten and drunk; the owner replied that Jess was not eating but was drinking a lot of water. Peter did not examine Jess or take her temperature. He supplied Jess's owner with some non-steroidal anti-inflammatories and suggested that Jess be presented to the clinic again on the Monday.

On Sunday morning Jess died, and on Monday morning Peter found himself with an irate client demanding his money back and the medical records as he intended to report the matter to the Veterinary Surgeons Board. During the week that followed, the board requested Jess's medical records and the veterinarians were asked to meet with the Board individually. The outcomes were: Jim's record keeping and physical examination were satisfactory, but given that the X-ray machine was not functioning, and that he was suspicious of pyometra, Jim should have immediately referred the case to another clinic, or even better to an emergency centre. Peter received a much more serious misconduct charge and was asked to produce information about record-keeping procedures as well as his approach to physical examination and diagnosis. The Veterinary Surgeons Board found that he had failed to examine and provide adequate veterinary care for his patient. For 2 weeks Peter thought he would lose his Registration Licence to practise as a veterinarian and he became depressed. He continued to make mistakes and, although his registration was not revoked, it really knocked him back. Peter began talking about retiring and selling the practice. Marge supported Peter during this time, encouraging him to stay and not lose faith over this situation. Marge knows that if Peter sells, she would be the first to go. It would be difficult for her to find another position as she had not 'up-skilled' by undertaking further training.

Keeping up to date with the competition

For years NVC has opened at 9 a.m. and closed at 5 p.m. Monday to Friday, and on Saturdays opened at 9 a.m. and closed at 11 a.m. However, clients of the new demographic are now asking for earlier drop-off times and later pick-up times, but the principal vet, Peter, refuses to extend opening hours. This causes friction at NVC and some staff start earlier (unpaid) to meet clients' needs. The competing veterinary clinics open at 7.30 a.m. and close at 8.00 p.m., allowing working professionals to access the clinic before or after work. Appointments at the competitor clinics are scheduled 30 minutes apart, allowing time for the care factor and attention to detail. The competing veterinary clinics also open the door for their clients and take cats in carriers to a quiet part of the waiting room away from dogs. The competing clinics have nurses working in a team with the veterinarian for consultations. The two competing practices appear to be busy, employing veterinarians that are attracting a younger, more vibrant clientele because of their special interest in birds, exotics and pocket pets. They are also offering wellness packages to encourage clients to pre-purchase a 12-month preventative health plan, and this includes pet insurance.

Time for an upgrade?

Dr Jim Chew is currently a little disgruntled and frustrated at the calibre of NVC's orthopaedic equipment. He believes there is a gap in the market for an orthopaedic service that would support the surrounding practices. He is confident he could fill this gap, but NVC's current equipment and facilities are poor. Upgrading the equipment alone would require an investment of $50 000.

Table 15.9 Benchmarking report – customized

	Min.	Poorest practice	O'Connor	Best of practices	Max.	Median	Average	Std dev.	Rel. pos.
Profitability KPIs									
Return on sales	5%	5%	17.2%	31%	31%	23%	20%	8%	50%
Inventory turnover	6.1	9.6	6.84	9.1	15.2	9.3	10.0	3.1	16%
Days in stock	24	38	53	40	59	39	40	11	88%
Productivity KPIs									
Full-time equivalent vets	2	2.5	2.5	2.5	4.6	2.5	2.6	0.7	42%
Average revenue per vet	$323 759	$323 759	$379 605	$417 566	$489 518	$379 605	$398 050	$54 738	37%
Medical revenue per vet	$279 964	$279 964	$378 802	$416 682	$488 081	$379 665	$380 278	$58 674	49%
Average TransCharge(ATC)	$40.96	$58.52	$82.78	$91.06	$91.06	$72.93	$71.43	$13.77	80%
Medical ATC	$37.58	$50.61	$82.61	$90.87	$90.87	$71.35	$69.02	$15.93	80%
Annual no. of trans/FTE	4 586	5 532	4 586	4 586	8 347	5 532	5 736	1 246	18%
Active clients per vet	850	1 005	1 290	1 290	1 561	1 290	1 228	197	62%
New clients/year/vet	112	254	347	258	427	268	295	103	69%
Annual transactions/client	3.6	5.5	3.6	3.6	9.8	4.4	4.9	1.8	24%
Annual revenue per client	$268	$322	$294	$324	$402	$322	$328	$40	20%
Cost-control KPIs									
Drug/medical supply costs as % of rev.	18.3%	23.80%	30.66%	24%	31.8%	27.6%	26.0%	4.0%	69%
Lab costs as % of revenue	0.2%	1.50%	1.9%	1.80%	2.5%	1.9%	1.8%	0.6%	60%
Retail prod. exp. % of rev.	0.1%	n/a	0.2%	0.14%	7.8%	0.2%	2.0%	3.0%	28%
Non-vet wages % of rev.	9.0%	n/a	12.0%	11%	29.0%	12.0%	14.8%	6.7%	34%
Rent-lease building as % of revenue	3.8%	7.00%	5.5%	7%	9.0%	7.0%	6.8%	1.8%	75%
Total costs as % of revenue	69.0%	95%	80.0%	69%	95.0%	77.0%	80.0%	8.3%	50%

Note: All practices have no owner compensation in the calculations, and VET FTE have 1 FTE owner for this benchmarking group. This is only relevant to the ratio 'Return on sales'.

Peter has suggested that Jim prepare a projection for the next 24 months in order to justify the outlay for orthopaedic equipment. As cash flow is poor, leasing the equipment would be the most likely financing option. Peter argues that there may be other priorities to be addressed, such as the practice's outdated software system, before new orthopaedic equipment could be considered.

The veterinary specific software records client details, history and financial transactions. However, the software is old and it is difficult to run any detailed reports. Marge, the practice manager, just produces the basic essentials for the accountant, and client reminders are left until the last minute – that is, if they are printed and sent at all.

At times Peter has discussed cutting back on veterinary clinical commitments and increasing the time he spends on the business. Earlier in the year, he had produced a budget to determine the actual running costs of the business. At the time of producing this budget, debts such as taxation fines and superannuation payments were not factored in. When these elements are included, the business appears to have no money to spare; things are going to be very tight financially this year but Peter thinks he can trade out of the situation (see Tables 15.2, 15.3, 15.4 and Figure 15.1).

Peter and Jim hurriedly submitted data to a practice benchmarking service whose annual survey is just about to close. This will help them see how the practice is performing compared to other similar veterinary practices around the country. The results came back quickly and highlighted potential for 'tuning' the NVC (see Tables 15.8 and 15.9).

The challenge ahead

From Peter's perspective, he needs a 5-year plan towards retirement. However, this does not necessarily mean he has to continue running the practice on a day-to-day basis; rather, he would continue to enjoy an income, doing part-time practice along with some travel. For Jim, the opportunity to own the practice is in the back of his mind. An alternative is to simply help improve the practice's financial performance so he would get a substantially increased income. This would enable Jim to earn sufficient income to build assets outside of the practice and enjoy his profession (especially if he could build a surgery caseload and have good equipment). As Jim prepares to sit down with Peter to discuss the best way forward for Northington, he starts to think about all the changes that will need to be made, and the significant investment that will be required to turn the practice around. Reflecting on all the practice data he has gathered up, he starts to wonder whether he can actually convince Peter to hand over the reins to enable him to take control.

Acknowledgements

This case study is fictitious. All persons, buildings, locations, and data used in this case study are not those of any real facility. Several of RxWorks Veterinary Practice Management Software reports have inspired the layout of some of the tables.

Parasol Kennels: innovative animal housing

16

Christopher J. Brown   Jane Taylor

CHAPTER OVERVIEW

This case is designed to help veterinary students explore innovation and sustainability within the broader veterinary and related sectors. The business upon which this particular case focuses is situated within a traditionally conservative construction subsector: animal housing. The study highlights an entrepreneurial small business that has achieved a great deal since its inception. It also amplifies the challenges the business has faced (and continues to face) in its bid to expand both within and beyond the UK market. In 2011, Parasol's approximate annual turnover for the entire group was £2.5 million. Its main offices and manufacturing facility are in Crediton, mid Devon, but an office also exists in Wolverhampton. Currently seven staff members (five full-time and two part-time) are employed. It is Parasol's intention to increase the number of employees to ten by the end of 2013. The organization comprises three company directors who are responsible for management, finance and operations; a RIBA chartered architect; a design and technical manager; and a marketing consultant.

LEARNING OUTCOMES

After reading this case study, students will be able to:
- Appreciate the importance of innovation and product quality within a small growing business.
- Understand some of the challenges facing a small business within the wider veterinary-related sector in its efforts to export.
- Apply business concepts to suggest how the particular company depicted in this case study might exploit the new market opportunities they have identified.

Introduction

Colin and Diana Taylor formed Parasol Kennels in 1992. The company was named after the innovative design and development of a circular kennel for Wood Green Animal Shelters, a leading animal charity specializing in dog and cat welfare. The 'Parasol Kennel' was registered as a unique design that same year. This innovative animal housing system was created in response to the Universities Federation for Animal Welfare's (UFAW) collaborative research project needs, primarily reducing stress in animals, particularly those housed for long periods. It was the social concern of the animal that was of utmost importance, but Parasol's solution had many other advantages, both in differentiating itself in the marketplace and in delivering other animal welfare benefits.

In its first year, two other modular 'Parasol Kennels' were built at the Lothian Animal Welfare Centre for the Scottish Society for the Prevention of Cruelty to Animals (SSPCA) in Balerno, near Edinburgh. This was the first example in this market of using a pre-assembled modular building system with pre-finished materials/surfaces, making transport and site erection very quick and easy. Other benefits included enhanced kennel hygiene; appreciably reduced construction, maintenance and cleaning costs; abridged noise emission; and significant energy conservation.

Other animal charities including the RSPCA and Dog's Trust, followed by Revenue and Customs, who appointed Parasol to develop a rolling programme of nine kennel projects around the UK, placed orders for Parasol's modular animal housing

© 2014, Elsevier Ltd.

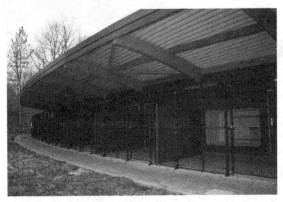

Figure 16.1 • Individual kennel pods

system. In 2003, the UK Ministry of Defence (MOD) placed the first of many orders for the Parasol modular animal housing system. Twelve kennel schemes have since been completed, and in 2010 Parasol designed and manufactured individual kennel 'pods' for the Société pour Protection des Animaux in Paris (Figure 16.1). Today, Parasol Kennels is the preferred supplier for the UK Border Agency (UKBA) and of the MOD dog housing needs. Key to this success is that Parasol's kennels exceed animal welfare regulations and comply with the MOD 'JSP315 Scale 14 requirements for Service Animals'.

The UK animal housing market

The animal housing market within the UK is very fragmented. Few animal housing construction companies offer products that meet current legislation. This is particularly the case within the private and commercial kennel sectors, which consist of boarding kennels, training establishments and dog breeders. Businesses compete in this particular marketplace by providing low-cost kennel solutions, often resulting in a lower-quality product. Many are constructed using low-grade steel for frames and wooden walls, which are no longer accepted by government, military, animal charities and animal welfare. Such materials are deemed short-lived and unhygienic.

Not-for-profit organizations rely entirely upon funding and charitable donations, so budgets for animal housing and ancillary buildings are tightly controlled. With the additional pressures of economic restrictions, design solutions are expected not only to satisfy the well-being of the animals, but also need to be highly efficient, cost effective and sustainable. The same applies to commercial projects for government departments such as the MOD and the UKBA; these organizations now demand compliance with BREEAM and DREAM standards, which require 'Excellent' ratings for sustainability, energy saving and adaptability. Investment in alternative and renewable energy resources is something currently being encouraged by both the government and a number of businesses throughout the UK, the great advantage being shorter-term returns on investment (ROI), often less than 5 years.

Those involved in animal housing within the public sector (PS) are exceptionally knowledgeable about the operational side of managing a kennel complex and the importance of animal welfare. It is their duty to maximize a professional working or service dog's potential in terms of performance, and keep veterinary expenses to a minimum. A fully trained detection dog, for example, is valued at around £25 k (Griffiths, 2012). Like humans, dogs will thrive and perform their tasks better and for longer if they are happily and suitably housed. So, in addition to their individual exercise and sleep compartments, access needs to be provided between all the exercise areas to allow the dogs to socialize.

Parasol Kennels considers itself as one of the innovative leaders of animal housing solutions in this fragmented marketplace, as co-founder and managing director Colin Taylor explains:

> We don't have too much direct competition and we are already ahead of the game, but in a business where you can't patent a building, you have to be always innovating to ensure you stay ahead.

The majority of the buyers of animal housing solutions today not only want the buildings to address animal welfare, but also expect them to address the issues and challenges of sustainability, energy saving and adaptability.

Parasol's business model and involvement in the UK animal housing market

Parasol Kennels invests substantially in design, research and development. The reason for doing so is to ensure that its animal housing systems are of premium quality, performing to the best of their ability, and are sold at the most competitive price. In fact this is the basis for its business model. As innovation is at the heart of everything it does, Parasol reacts quickly to changing market conditions and requirements,

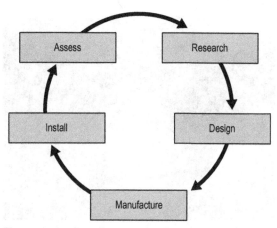

Figure 16.2 • Excellence model: Parasol's culture

while being proactive in inventing new solutions to help solve difficult customer challenges. Learning is at the core of Parasol's culture (Figure 16.2); continual assessment of customer needs initiates product innovation and enhancement, delivering business and customer value. For example, when one of Parasol's military buildings was independently measured by DREAM – the world's leading design and assessment method for sustainable buildings – it achieved the performance rating of 'Excellent'.

One member of the Parasol team – RIBA chartered architect John Flavell – has witnessed considerable change within the animal housing market, and has been hugely influential in the design of kennel projects in the private and public sectors. John has worked with regional and national animal charities, boarding establishments, the MOD and UKBA. He believes that all kennels should now be sustainable and manufactured to the highest level of quality, which would mean everyone concerned adhering to a completely new set of guidelines:

> The passing of the Animal Welfare Act 2006 was a major step forward in the protection of animals, but was a missed opportunity to update the guidelines under the Act. Parasol had an opportunity to provide leadership, and gained some competitive advantage, but unless there is more effective enforcement of the current regulations, progress in improving animal housing in general will remain slow. The responsibility for policing the rules remains with the Local Authority Environmental departments.

John would now like to see a Kennel Management Course being established in the country and for it to become a mandatory prerequisite for the handling of all dogs.

Parasol's reactive solutions

The welfare and well-being of an animal has been a social influence for kennel design and manufacturing for many years. Parasol offers both a parasol-shaped circular kennel and a linear version. Traditionally, the MOD and UKBA prefer linear kennels, whereas a number of regional and national animal charities select the circular layout. Both have sustainable advantages, but the parasol-shaped design has slightly more (Figure 16.3).

The Parasol kennel design has only been modified slightly throughout the years. The sizes of the sleep and exercise areas have been increased, and the entrance way and central services core now provide more valuable space for kitchen and food preparation activities. It is designed so that each segment contains a sleep area from which access can be gained into the central core. The central core provides a storage area for bedding and cleaning materials. The short distance between each segment and central core has a distinct advantage over the linear type. It is only 3 m to travel to any of the 15 sleep compartments from the centre of the circular kennel, whereas with a linear layout it can be up to 30 m.

Considerably less time is needed in the handling and management of the dogs within a parasol-shaped kennel as opposed to the linear version, and in some instances fewer staff are required. It is the shape that makes the difference. The entrance to each segment can be fitted out as a small preparation area from which food can be distributed to the external exercise area. But each of the 16 segments does not have to be used as sleep quarters: they are versatile enough to be used for something else, like a dog grooming room, for example (Figure 16.4).

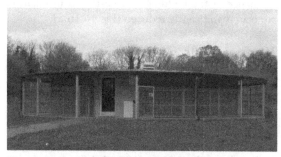

Figure 16.3 • Parasol designed animal housing

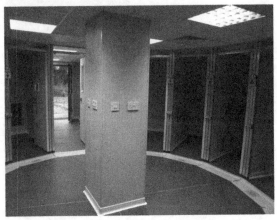

Figure 16.4 • Parasol internal arrangement of the sleeping and core areas

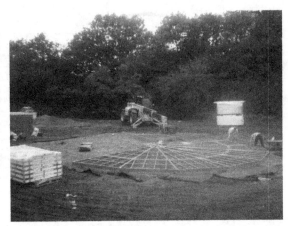

Figure 16.5 • Parasol modular floor

Parasol's proactive solutions

Some examples of the product innovations that regularly enhance Parasol's animal housing systems are outlined below.

Kennel floors

What became evident on a number of projects was that the concrete floors constructed by site ground workers did not comply with the close tolerances required for the effective installation of a Parasol kennel. If the concrete slab was uneven or not accurately measured, the erection of pre-fabricated panels became very difficult. It meant that time was wasted in the lining and levelling of the wall panels, and proved to be an inefficient and costly exercise. Parasol invented a new solution that entailed the creation of insulated internal partitions with slopes at the base – allowing for falls into drainage channels and gulleys to work properly – supported on a galvanized steel support framework fixed down or attached via anchor points. Besides improving the energy performance of the building, site costs and installation time are significantly reduced (Figure 16.5).

Kennel walls and roof

Parasol originally used cement particle board (CPB) for the internal walls of their kennels, and a sectional moulded glass-reinforced plastic (GRP) for the roof. Subsequent moulded roofs were used on similar buildings elsewhere. However, disadvantages soon emerged regarding the use of CPB. It was very heavy

to handle during the manufacturing process and at installation stage. It also proved not to be as thermally efficient as other modern sheeting/cladding. In addition, the moulded GRP roof was not that stable or easy to apply. A new, more sustainable and environmentally efficient alternative was found. It came in the form of a lightweight, hygienic, insulated sandwich panel using the latest adhesives and sealants for reliable bonding during manufacturing and at installation. These panels are perfect for creating wall and roof panels, with features including hygienic hard-wearing surfaces, and can be finished in various textures containing sound-attenuating cores that are both lightweight, transportable and easily installed on site (Figure 16.6).

Kennel ventilation and heating

Addressing another important animal welfare issue – heating and ventilation within the animal housing – has resulted in Parasol developing its own unique product. Kennels require between 10 and 12 volumetric air changes per hour. Conventional heating systems such as radiators and electric convectors, if used in these environments, would need to operate constantly, and heat would then be wasted. Running extractor fans on a prolonged basis is not only extremely costly but also creates noise disturbance to both dogs and staff. Parasol use a 'Venturi' effect to generate constant natural ventilation through the use of one medium-power extractor. The extractor system can be set on a timer and controlled by a humidistat and other air quality sensors. Heating for the dogs is provided by infrared radiant heaters which only heat the dogs and their

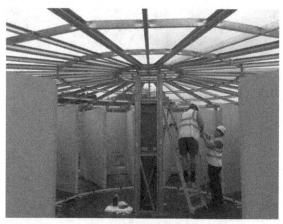

Figure 16.6 • New wall composite design

surrounding surface, and not the air around them. The solution means that there is a reduced risk of losing clean air or heat, and therefore no wastage, which leads to cost savings.

Animal welfare

Parasol's comprehensive knowledge of animal welfare prompted it to select a different material for the prevention of animal injury. It learnt that kennels using mesh panels quite often resulted in a dog hurting its claws when jumping up against them. Parasol typically uses vertical bars instead of mesh, so dog claw injuries are dramatically reduced. Other benefits include reduced veterinary bills and lower animal stress levels. Steel bars are also much easier and quicker to clean and maintain.

Parasol's network: acquiring knowledge and competences

Parasol's product and business development has resulted from its active use of outside communities and support agencies to understand market needs as well as the technologies and knowledge required for developing product solutions. Equally, during the design and installation phases of each project, Parasol has worked with several major consultancy companies in overall procurement and delivery, ensuring cost and time deliverables.

Via the internet, the business has been able to learn about and introduce new technologies from Europe and the USA, create new relationships with suppliers of modern sheeting and insulation materials

sharing the same vision and, in general on a global level, exchange ideas. This phenomenon has resulted in Parasol sourcing the GRP facing sheet on the insulated panels from manufacturers in Germany, and obtaining acoustic insulation used within the composite roof cladding from Belgium.

Within the UK, Parasol has created a network of specialists who help the business to develop new techniques and competences in manufacturing for its innovative panels and product solutions. These partnerships have facilitated the introduction of modern materials and installation techniques, particularly those involving modular fittings and pre-wiring capabilities within pre-fabricated modular walls.

Parasol also has strong affiliations with approval bodies and associations. The Building Research Establishment (BRE) assesses and evaluates the performance of the insulated panels they use for their modular systems. In addition, the National Energy Action (NEA) Trust has enrolled the services of the business since 2006 to create measurable energy-efficient solutions for the prevention of fuel wastage, a system now approved by OFGEM (Office of Gas and Electricity Markets). This is another part of the business which, while not discussed here, demonstrates the application of the design of animal housing to other areas, such as social housing.

Future growth and development

Now that Parasol's products have been fully tried and tested in the UK, the company is keen to explore overseas markets. However, Parasol still needs to determine which markets it should leverage first, and then identify those that best match its unique competences.

Using the services of the UK Trade and Investment (UKTI) Department, Parasol has taken advantage of the 'Passport to Export' scheme that offers businesses assistance with their export strategy. The business has already received interest from organizations in Ireland, Belgium and New Zealand, but with the additional help of UKTI it could significantly expand its global reach to other prospective markets – particularly those with substantial military and security operations.

Meanwhile, in the UK, Parasol has identified an opportunity for a 'flat-pack' single-kennel solution amongst the domestic and smaller private and commercial animal housing operators. Parasol's MD,

Colin, describes it as 'the one stop shop kennel'. Being quick and easy to install, relocatable, easy to export in a container, made using high-quality materials that enhance hygiene and acoustics, and self-ventilating will all be important elements for success. However, there is already considerable competition in this market, and Parasol will need to decide whether its particular competences relating to design and building kennels really deliver a unique selling point (USP).

A further area for potential development is the diversification of Parasol's modular ancillary buildings into new sectors such as medical, veterinary, education and border security. As the ancillary buildings offer the same sustainable, energy-saving and adaptable benefits, this could constitute an attractive proposition to those outside of the kennels arena. Using a modular structure and a type of construction designed to provide temporary accommodation or disaster housing within high-risk global areas threatened by earthquakes and other such natural disasters could be another sector that Parasol could potentially target.

Interestingly, one particular area of the business that is developing momentum is the provision of alternative energy systems to support the remote locations of some animal housing projects (Figure 16.7). What initially started out as a need to provide security of supply for the energy needs of these remote projects has now developed into an opportunity to supply energy system packages as stand-alone systems. The first system to go live was at the animal housing for the MOD at Brize Norton. Parasol now integrates renewable solutions within its modular building schemes. These include wind turbines and masts, air source heat pumps, and future photo-voltaic (PV) designs to create a modular 'sun and wind' energy system. Parasol is still undertaking extensive product testing to ensure that its claims for power generation can be supported by strong empirical field data, but the opportunity exists both in the animal housing marketplace and beyond.

Clearly, there are several expansion opportunities open to the company to enable it to break into the global export marketplace. Reflecting on the various options, Parasol's MD, Colin, fully appreciates that he will need to identify those opportunities that offer the best fit with the business's competences and resources, while at the same time offering the greatest potential for growth. Long-term success in the global market will ultimately depend on the strength of its export strategy.

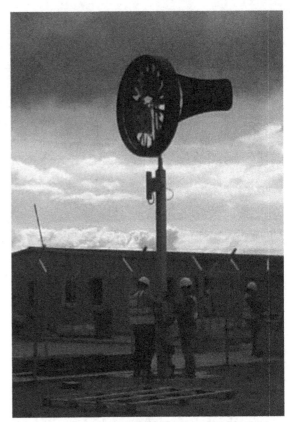

Figure 16.7 • Parasol's energy systems solutions

Appendix: regulations within the UK and Northern Ireland

The Universities Federation for Animal Welfare (UFAW) has always promoted the importance of animal welfare, and continuously investigates, through a scientific approach, ways of assessing what matters to animals, their welfare and how to improve their quality of life:

> Ensuring good welfare is about more than ensuring good health. Animal welfare is about the quality of animals' lives: their feelings. It is now widely agreed, although it was not always so, that many species are sentient – they have capacity to feel pain and distress, they can suffer and, conversely, be aware of pleasant feelings – and that this matters morally. (Importance of Science, 2012)

UFAW works in conjunction with other organizations and individuals such as animal keepers, scientists, veterinarians and lawyers to ensure knowledge is enhanced.

The Animal Welfare Act 2006 contains the general laws relating to animal welfare, and states that it is an offence to cause unnecessary suffering to any animal (DEFRA, 2012a, 2012b). Unlike previous legislation, it applies to all animals on common land, and contains a Duty of Care. This means that anyone responsible for an animal must take reasonable steps to ensure the animal's needs are met and that it does not suffer.

The Animal Boarding Establishments Act 'regulates the keeping of boarding establishments for animals; and for purposes connected therewith' (http://www.legislation.gov.uk/ukpga/1963/43). It requires businesses where the boarding of animals is being carried out to obtain a licence from the local authority. In 1993, The Chartered Institute of Environmental Health (CIEH) published comprehensive guidance and model licence conditions to ensure that a consistent approach was maintained in the issuing of licences and the enforcement of the legislation by local authorities (CIEH Working Party Report, October 1995). But following the publication of the conditions, it became apparent that there were a number of inconsistencies and discrepancies. This resulted in a working group consisting of CIEH, the Association of District Councils (ADC), British Veterinary Association (BVA), British Small Animal Veterinary Association (BSAVA), Feline Advisory Bureau (FAB) and Pet Trade and Industry Association (PTIA) meeting to consider changes in the format of the conditions to improve readability,

interpretation and consistent application. The 'Working Party Report' was published in 1995.

There was legal confusion and a lack of regulation for security dogs until a new British Standard – BS8517-1 – for general-purpose security dogs was introduced in 2009. The standard now prevents anyone from setting up as a trainer or supplier of guard dogs, and includes requirements such as security dogs undergoing training with a minimum of 50 guided learning hours. However, the BS8517-1 is a code of practice and not a law, albeit a very useful one, and should legal authorities become involved they will take the view that security dog handlers should be working to the standard. From a legal perspective, the most useful piece of legislation regarding the well-being of a security dog is the Health and Safety at Work Act 1974.

The British military currently use their own 'scales' – JSP314 Scales 1, 13, 14, 18 and 40 – for professional service working dogs, which comply with the Animal Welfare Act 2006, and with the Model Licence Conditions and Guidance for Dog Boarding Establishments under the Animal Boarding Establishments Act 1963. It is taking the military some time to bring their kennels and amenities buildings up to the exact requirements of the regulations, and in some instances kennels installed not that long ago now have to be replaced with more efficient, portable and sustainable solutions in order to meet the high expectations of animal welfare.

References

DEFRA, 2012a. Legislation (accessed 31.07.12). Available:http://www.defra.gov.uk/food-farm/animals/welfare/on-farm/legislation/

DEFRA, 2012b. Protecting pets from cruelty (accessed 31.07.12).

Available: http://www.defra.gov.uk/wildlife-pets/pets/cruelty/html

Griffiths, J., 2012. Spotlight: man's best friend (accessed 31.07.12). Available: http://www.iosh.co.uk/news_and_events/connect/58_guard_dogs.aspx.html

Importance of Science, 2012 (accessed 06.11.12). Available: http://www.ufaw.org.uk/animal-welfare.php

Index

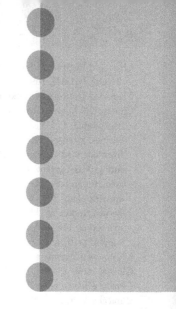

Note: Page numbers followed by *b* indicate boxes, *f* indicate figures, *t* indicate tables and *np* indicate footnotes.